Boari Bladder-Flap Procedure

Single Surgical Procedures 7

A Colour Atlas of

Boari Bladder-Flap Procedure

James G. Gow

W DE G

Walter de Gruyter · Berlin · New York 1984

James G. Gow MD, Ch. M, FRCS; Consultant Urologist (Emeritus), Liverpool Area Health Authority (Teaching), Past President of the Section of Urology of the Royal Society of Medicine

Original Publishers: Wolfe Medical Publications Ltd., · London
Exclusive co-publishers for the Federal Republic of Germany and Austria: Walter de Gruyter & Co., Genthiner Strasse 13, D-1000 Berlin 30. 1984.

Printed by Royal Smeets Offset b.v., Weert, Netherlands

Cover design: Rudolf Hübler

General Editor, Wolfe Surgical Atlases:
William F. Walker, DSc, ChM, FRCS (Eng.), FRCS (Edin.), FRS (Edin.)

CIP-Kurztitelaufnahme der Deutschen Bibliothek

Gow, James G.:
A colour atlas of boari bladder-flap procedure / James G. Gow. – Berlin; New York: de Gruyter, 1984.
(Single surgical procedures; 7)
ISBN 3-11-010032-0
ISBN 3-11-010033-9 (Subskr.-Pr.)
NE: GT

Contents

Introduction

Achille Boari, the Italian surgeon, first described the technique of ureterocystoplasty for reconstructive surgery of the lower ureter in 1894. He constructed a tube made from a pedicle bladder flap, to replace the lower ureter in a dog.

This technique was not used on man until 1930, when it was first reported by Baidin. The second recorded case on man was reported by Ockerblad and Carlson, who described the technique for ureterovesical fistula in 1939.

The most comprehensive early paper was by Cukier in 1966. This paper described the results of 63 operations carried out at the Couvelaire Clinic. It also pointed out the good results achieved in cases suffering from tuberculosis and trauma, and the relatively poor results achieved in cases of malignancy.

It also underlined the superiority of the submucous tunnelling technique over end-to-end anastomosis, and stressed the improvement in results when splintage at the anastomotic site was abandoned. It is one of the most useful techniques in urology, and rescues the urologist time and time again.

The Boari flap may be single (**1a**). Occasionally two ureters have to be transplanted (**1b**). There is no fear of a bladder of permanently small capacity when two flaps are raised, although it may appear alarmingly small, because it will expand to an equivalent size as long as the trigone and detrusor muscle are not damaged by interstitial cystitis, irradiation or tuberculosis. Sometimes it is impossible to reimplant both ureters, because the gap between the normal ureter and the bladder is too wide to bridge. In this case a uretero-ureterostomy is carried out above the bladder and the ureter anastomosed to a single Boari flap (**1c**).

The commonest pathological conditions requiring a Boari reconstruction are:

Trauma

Operative:

a) Extensive ablative surgical techniques for cancer.
b) After gynaecological surgery.
c) Ureterovaginal fistulae.
d) Fibrosis after ureterolithotomy.
e) After vascular surgery on the aorta.

Inflammation:

a) Tuberculosis.
b) Bilharzia.
c) Involvement of the ureter in a pericolic abscess, secondary to diverticulitis.

Pelvic irradiation used especially for carcinoma of the cervix.

Megaureter.

Idiopathic dilatation of the lower end of the ureter.

Many urologists use a uretero-ureterostomy for some of these conditions, but the author is conscious of the negligible, but very real danger to the good ureter.

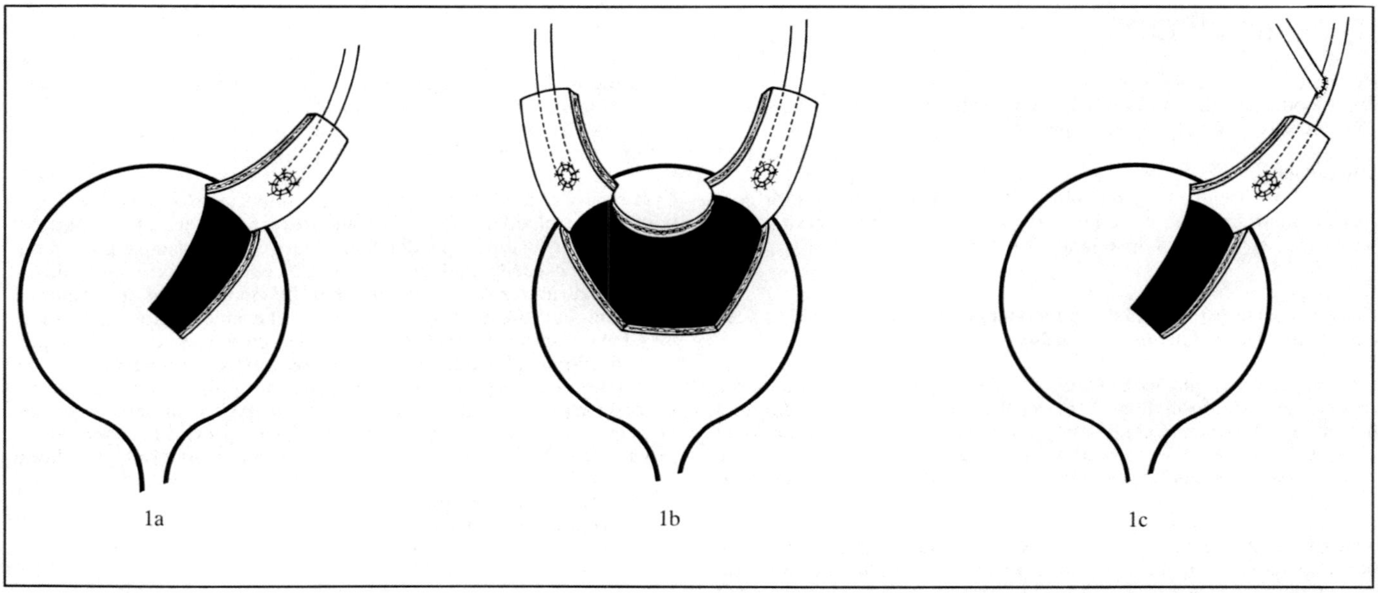

1a Single Boari flap.

1b Double Boari flap.

1c Single Boari flap with ureter-oureterostomy.

Investigations

Haematological and biochemical
Full blood count and differential, erythrocyte sedimentation rate, urea and electrolytes should be performed.

Microbiology
The urine is examined for red and white cells and is cultured for non-specific organisms and *M. tuberculosis*. If infection is present, it should be treated before the reimplantation is performed.

Radiology
Chest xray. This will reveal any pulmonary metastases if there has been a previous history of neoplastic disease.

Intravenous urography with or without tomography. This procedure will reveal essential information of the renal function and the condition of the ureter. A dynamic study using the image intensifier is important because it gives a better indication as to the extent of the disease, the peristaltic activity, the length of the stricture and the amount of fibrosis that may be present.

Retrograde pyelography. It may be necessary to use this procedure if the intravenous urogram does not give satisfactory information. This examination is again performed under direct vision using a bulb-ended catheter to introduce the contrast.

Percutaneous antegrade pyelography. This investigation may be necessary if an intravenous urogram fails and contrast will not pass up the ureter through a retrograde catheter. It may give essential information of the excretory pathways above an obstruction.

Radioisotope investigation. Renal scanning affords information of functioning renal tissue and can estimate the amount of renal function that a diseased kidney is contributing to the total renal function.

Ultrasound. This examination may reveal a secondary tumour in the liver and will show an enlarged kidney with a dilated pelvicalyceal system.

Computerised axial tomography. Masses in the pelvis will be shown with this technique. It will also confirm liver tumours and give in greater detail the dilatation of the pelvicalyceal system. It is rarely necessary before carrying out the Boari procedure.

Cystoscopy. A preliminary cystoscopy is important to assess the condition of the bladder. The following specific changes are important: bladder trabeculation, bladder outlet obstruction, bladder induration, and a small capacity bladder. If there is an acute tuberculous cystitis, a preliminary ureterostomy *in situ* may be necessary as a temporary expedient, because after five to six weeks of chemotherapy, the bladder may have improved sufficiently for a definitive procedure to be performed. When planning this procedure, certain factors have to be considered, because they often contribute towards poor results. These factors include previous irradiation of the pelvis, ureters which are dilated and require tapering, and multiple previous ureterovesical procedures which may have damaged the blood supply to the lower ureter.

The aims of the procedure must always be:

1. To preserve renal function.
2. To re-establish continuity of the lower ureter without reflux.

Preoperative preparation

If the reimplantation is necessary as a result of a tuberculous stricture, at least four weeks antituberculous treatment should be given before surgery, and this treatment must be continued without interruption until the course is completed. A lower urinary tract infection is treated with an appropriate antibiotic, which is continued during the postoperative period until the bladder catheter is removed. If there is a ureterovaginal fistula, a full vaginal preparation is carried out, and if the cause of the obstruction is inflammation secondary to diverticulitis, the bowel is prepared by means of a colonic lavage, followed by a povidine–iodine retention enema.

Technique

Before the operation is started an 18 Charrière–Foley catheter, with a 20ml balloon, is passed into the bladder and attached to a reservoir containing normal saline.

The best incision is a Pfannenstiel, with an extension into one or other iliac fossa, depending on whether one or two ureters are being re-implanted. The external internal oblique and transversalis muscles are incised, and the peritoneum gently reflected medially. It may be necessary to free the peritoneum from the superior and posterior surfaces of the bladder, but this is not necessary unless a flap of more than 12cm is required. With adequate preparation, mobilisation of the bladder should make it possible to bridge a ureteric gap of 16cm, and even this amount can be exceeded if the kidney is mobilised and brought down towards the pelvis.

The ureter is then mobilised. It should first be approached above the diseased area, so that a normal ureter can be followed to the point at which there is obvious damage. The superior vesical vessel is ligated on the side of the lesion; very occasionally it may be necessary to ligate the contralateral vessel to mobilise the bladder adequately. The bladder is then filled with saline and the flap is delineated with stay sutures.

Unlike a normal skin flap, because of the excellent blood supply to the bladder, the length of the flap may be much longer than the width, so that a precise flap can always be formed.

The flap is then cut. Vessels are either coagulated by diathermy under-run or ligated. If the flap is to extend over to the other side of the bladder, it is advisable to pass a large catheter, size 6, up the contralateral ureter, so that it can be easily felt when the extremity of the flap is being cut. However, the author has found this rarely necessary.

The ureter is implanted into the tunnel, which must be at least 5cm in length, and sutured, mucosa to mucosa, by interrupted 4.0 Dexon sutures. Some authorities suggest a cuff, but the author has never used this technique, because he does not feel that it has any advantage and only prolongs operating time.

Occasionally, if the ureter is fibrosed and thickened, it would be unnecessarily hazardous to attempt a submucous tunnel; in these cases, reflux has to be accepted. This situation is rare and usually occurs in cases of tuberculosis. The author, like Cukier, does not splint the anastomosis, and has never regretted this technique, although it is accepted that many surgeons would prefer to complete the anastomosis over a splint.

The bladder is closed in two continuous layers, using 3.0 Dexon. The ureter is sutured to the apex of the flap by a series of 4.0 or 5.0 Dexon, and the flap is then sutured to the psoas muscle.

The wound is closed in layers with an indwelling catheter and a drain down to the area of the anastomosis.

Because the indwelling urethral catheter will remain for seven or eight days, it is customary to give antibiotic cover until it is removed. The drain is taken out after four or five days.

Results

Most of the recorded results are for ureteric injuries. Konigsberg (1975) reported the results of this operation on 23 patients: 15 were satisfactory, but eight were considered poor. Of these eight, three had undergone irradiation, another had carcinoma of the bladder, which recurred in the flap, and four had some failure in technique. In two the flap was not fixed to the psoas muscle, and in the other two strictures reformed, probably as a result of too vigorous mobilisation of the tissue, and poor ureteric blood supply.

Thompson (1977) reported the results of 38 patients who were treated for ureteral injuries. In 25 patients a mucosa-to-mucosa anastomosis had to be carried out. It was noted that no deterioration in renal function was present, that the normal renal architecture had been maintained, and that the urine had not become infected. In this group, there were three failures – one as a result of continuation of retro-peritoneal fibrosis; one in which the bladder-flap procedure was a second attempt, and the third when a stent was used to drain the ureter.

Thompson also noticed that the bladder tube appeared eventually to conform more to ureteric appearance, and the narrow conduit from the ureter to the bladder will appear as though it was part of the ureter.

In the author's series of 47 (Table 1), most of the cases are caused by tuberculosis. However, there has been a change of pattern. In the paper (Gow, 1968) most of the tuberculous ureters were fibrotic, but since then most strictures have been with proximal ureteric dilatation; therefore it has been possible to perform a tunnel technique with occasional tapering. In 14 of the other 17 cases it was possible to use the tunnel technique. These results are shown in Table 2. The three cases of reflux occurred in the early cases, and are almost certainly caused by a tunnel that was too short.

Complications

Haemorrhage
This may be reactive or secondary. Reactionary haemorrhage occurs within 24 hours and comes either from the plexus of veins around the ureter, or from the bladder. Secondary haemorrhage, which usually occurs two to three weeks after surgery, is rarely seen.

Urinary fistula
This complication is rare if the bladder is sutured in two layers, and if the bladder is filled with fluid before closing the abdomen. It nearly always stops spontaneously.

Wound infection
Infection is always a possibility if there has been previous irradiation or pelvic infection. It can be reduced by the use of an appropriate antibiotic. It may lead to a keloid scar.

Ureteric stenosis
Stenosis usually occurs in a diseased fibrotic ureter. After surgery an intravenous urogram is performed in one month, and then at intervals according to the progress of the anastomosis.

Renal failure
This complication may occur if the ureter of a diseased kidney is reimplanted in an attempt to save the kidney.

Ruptured deep epigastic artery
A rare complication caused by too vigorous retraction.

Table 1 Author's series, indications for reconstruction in 47 patients.

Tuberculosis: Fibrous ureter	17
Stricture and dilatation	15
Injury to ureter during surgery	4
Involvement of ureter in pathological process	4
Ureterovaginal fistula	2
After gynaecological surgery	5

Table 2 Results of surgery in author's patients.

		Reflux	Reduction in hydronephrosis
Side to side anastomosis with hydronephrosis	20	19	16
Tunnel technique			
With hydronephrosis	16	2	13
Without hydronephrosis	11	1	—

Stage 1

1 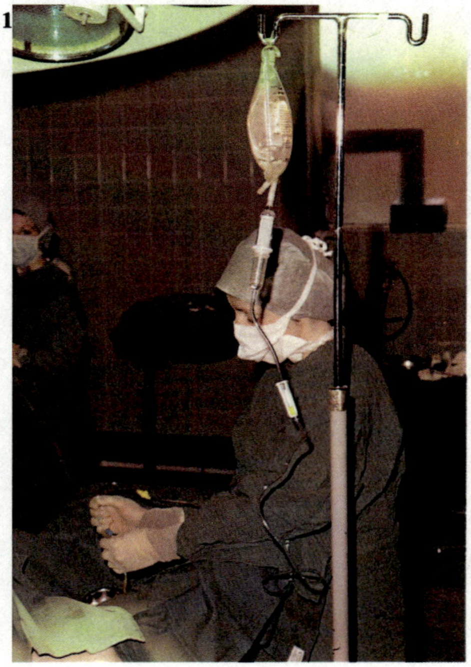

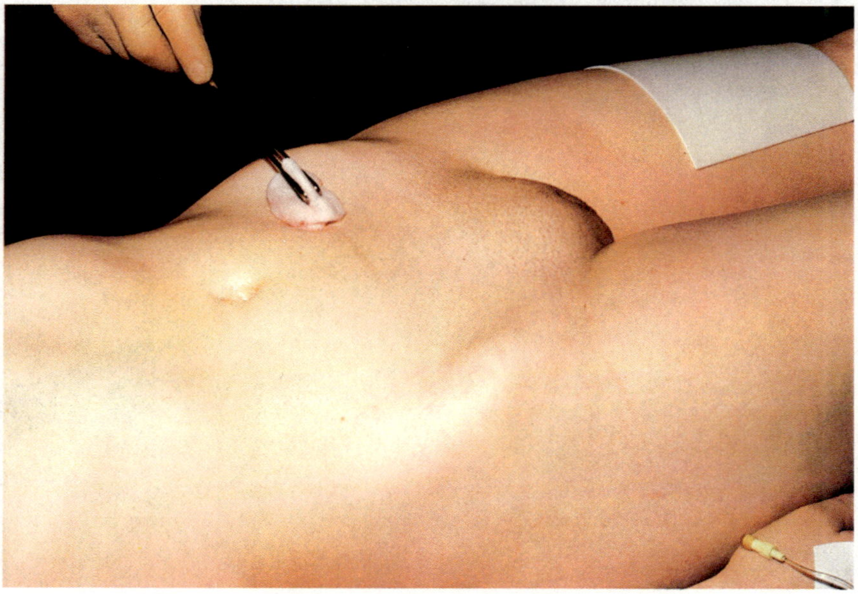 2

1 Before the patient is towelled up, the catheter is attached to a reservoir of normal saline. This reservoir is used to fill the bladder when the time has come for the Boari flap to be constructed, and just before closure to ensure there are no leaks.

2 The patient is placed in the supine position, with slight head-down tilt. Preparation is carried out with hibitane (chlorhexidine) spirit, although there are many other substances which are equally effective.

Note the adhesive diathermy pad, which is smoothly attached to the thigh, to reduce the chance of a diathermy burn.

3 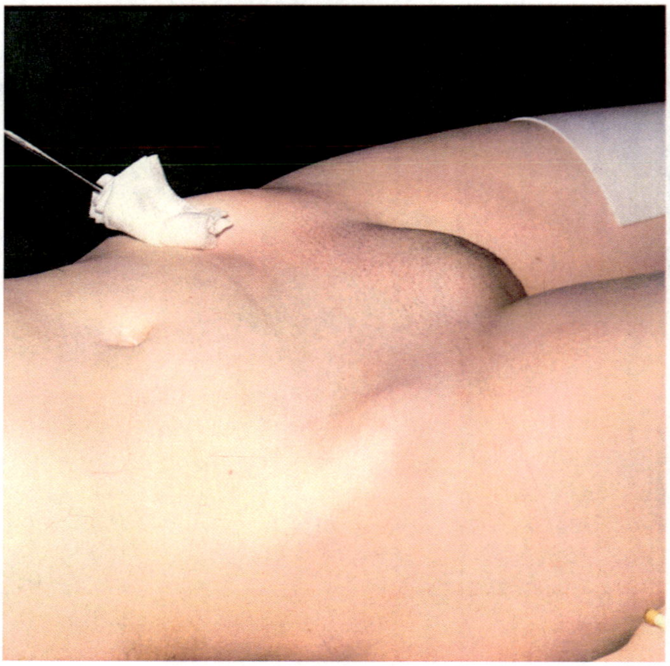

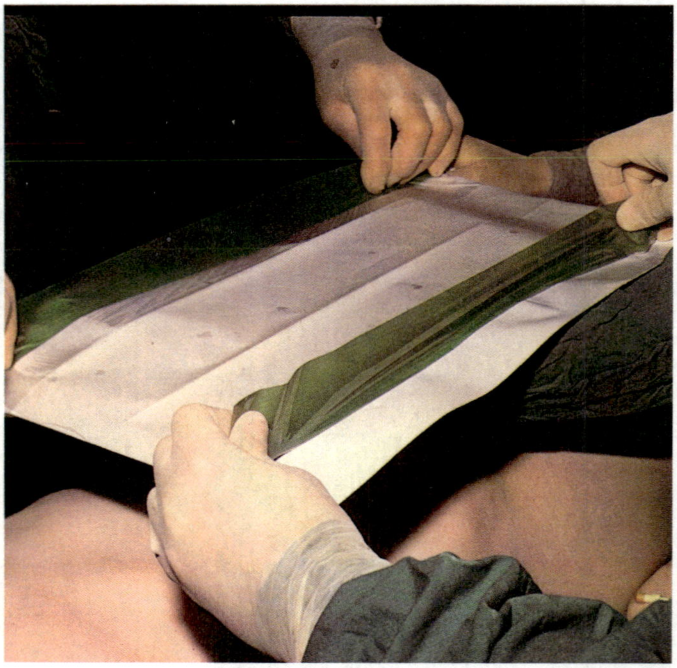 4

3 The skin is carefully dried, and then there is a short wait before the Op-site dressing is applied. Op-site is a polyurethane film with an adhesive. Polyurethane allows perspiration to pass through, but not bacteria. It can be left on for four to five days, and then it is removed, when the skin is normal. This adhesive dressing is comforting for the patient, reduces the incidence of infection, and gives admirable support to the skin in the first few days after surgery.

4 Stretching of the film after the removal of the protective backing.

5

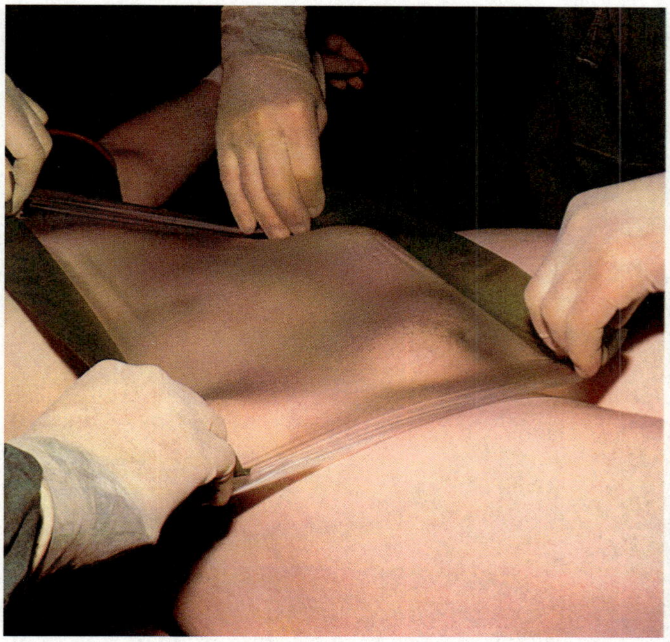

6

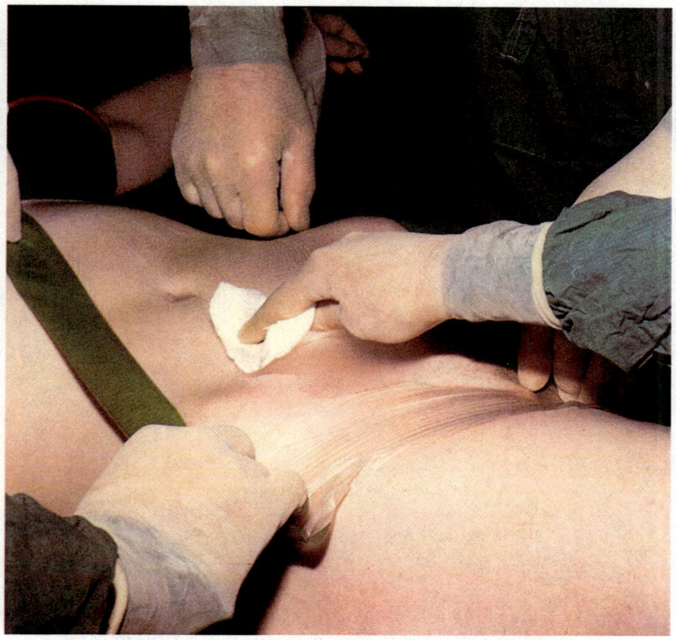

5 Application of the stretched film to the abdomen.

6 Final pressure with a swab or pack to achieve maximum adhesion.

7

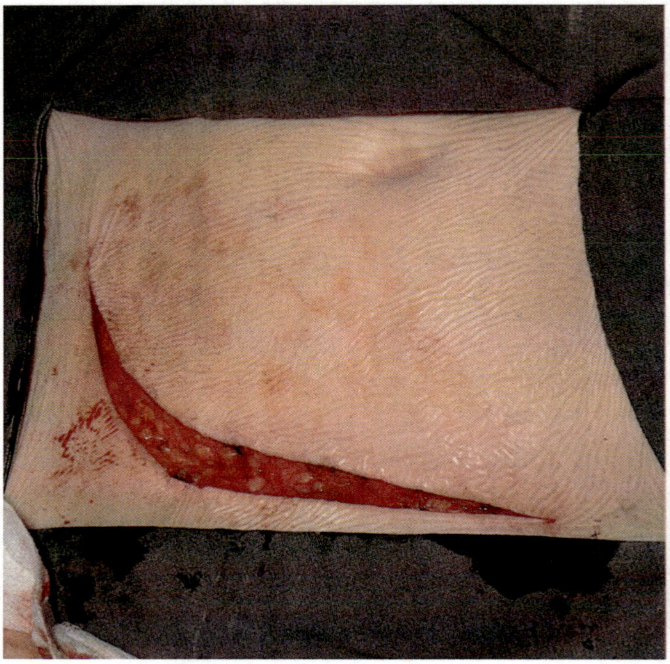

8

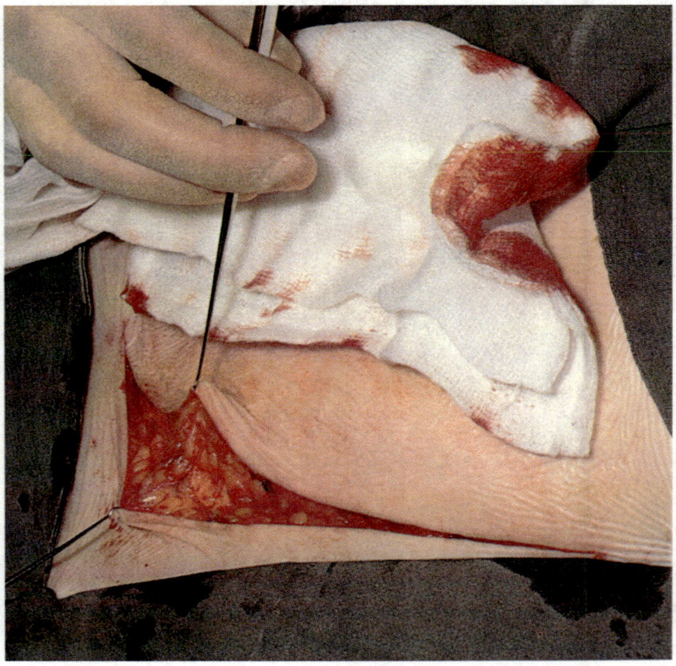

7 The incision is an extended Pfannenstiel. The depth of the first cut is to the rectus sheath and all superficial vessels are coagulated with diathermy. The extension is on the side on which the reimplantation is going to be carried out, and if it is bilateral the extension can easily be made into both iliac fossae.

Note the satisfactory adhesion of the Op-site to the wound edges. This only happens if the skin is dry and the Op-site is allowed to adhere before the incision is made.

8 Small sharp skin hooks, mainly used by plastic surgeons, are used to elevate the skin after the initial incision is made. This reduces trauma to the skin edges which might occur if larger instruments were used.

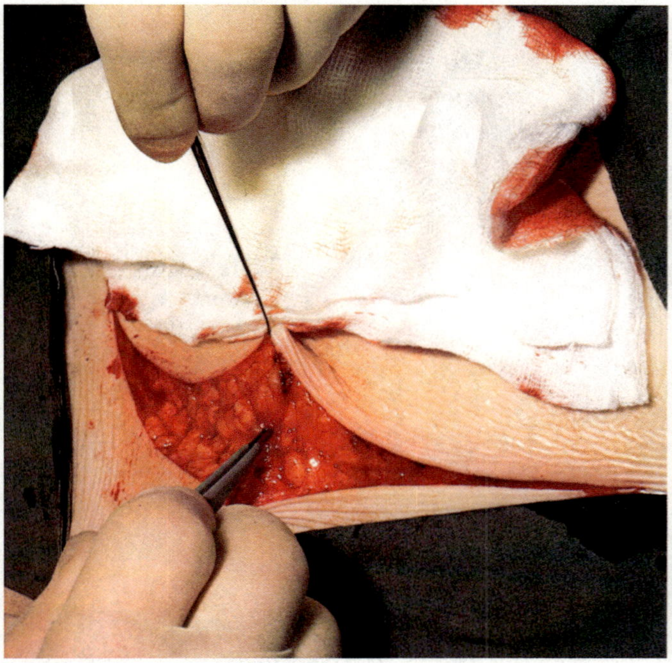

9 **Haemostasis is obtained by using a fine diathermy forceps.** Another method is to use fine forceps, either McIndoe or Gillies, and together with a diathermy needle or diathermy scalpel.

10

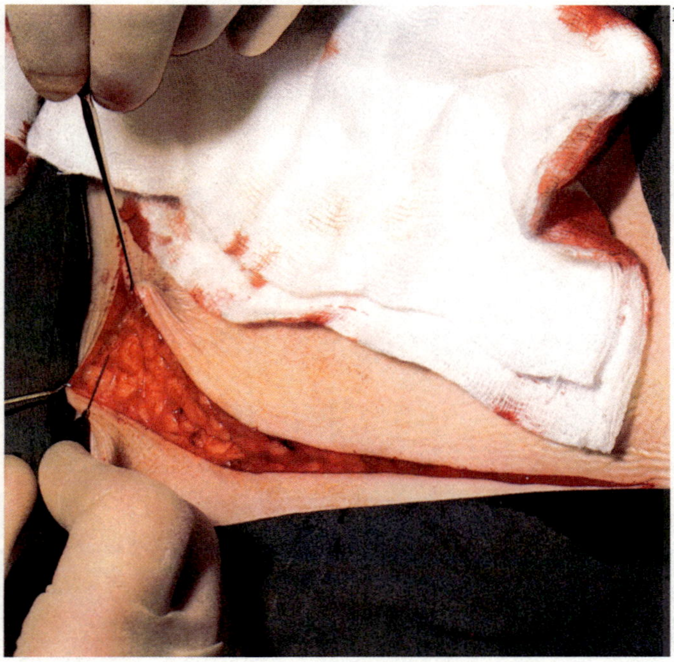

10 **After the skin incision is made**, the next layers are carefully dissected, using a fine diathermy needle. A scalpel is an attractive method, but the blood-loss is greater.

11 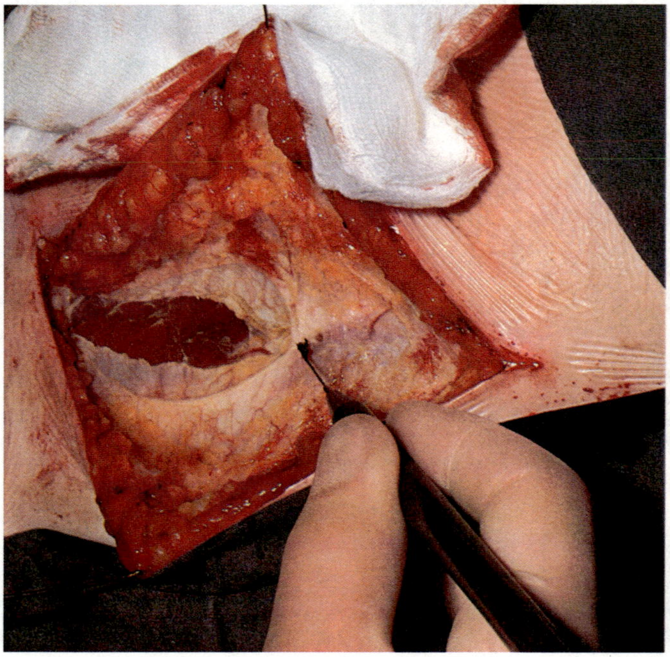

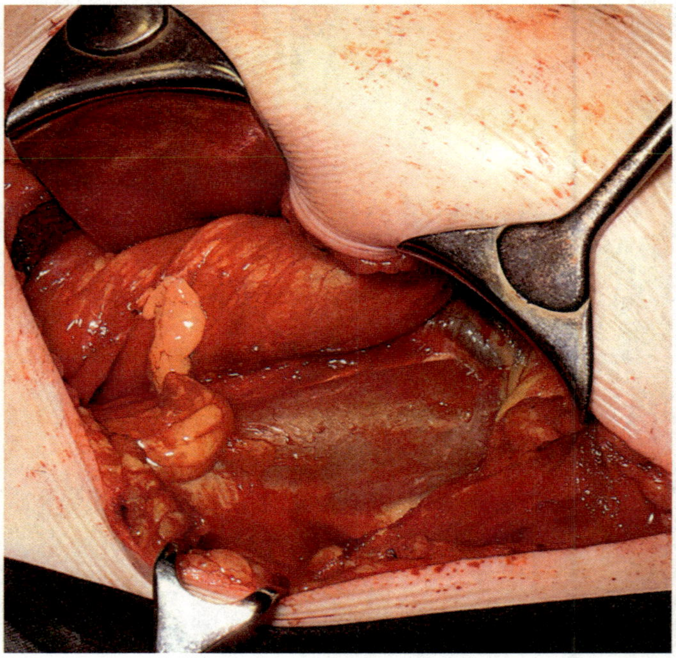 12

11 The external oblique is being dissected, and the aponeurosis can be seen joined to the muscle. The rectus sheath has also been identified and incised, and the rectus muscle can be seen clearly. Note the excellent exposure with the skin hooks, and again the good adhesion of the Op-site to the edges of the wound, even with extensive traction, which is necessary to obtain a satisfactory exposure.

12 After the external oblique, internal oblique and the rectus sheath are incised, the transversalis is carefully cut, and the peritoneum exposed. The peritoneum is then reflected medially, displaying the psoas muscle. (Note the plexus of veins close to the lower retractor, which can cause extensive haemorrhage unless retraction is gently and carefully carried out.)

13

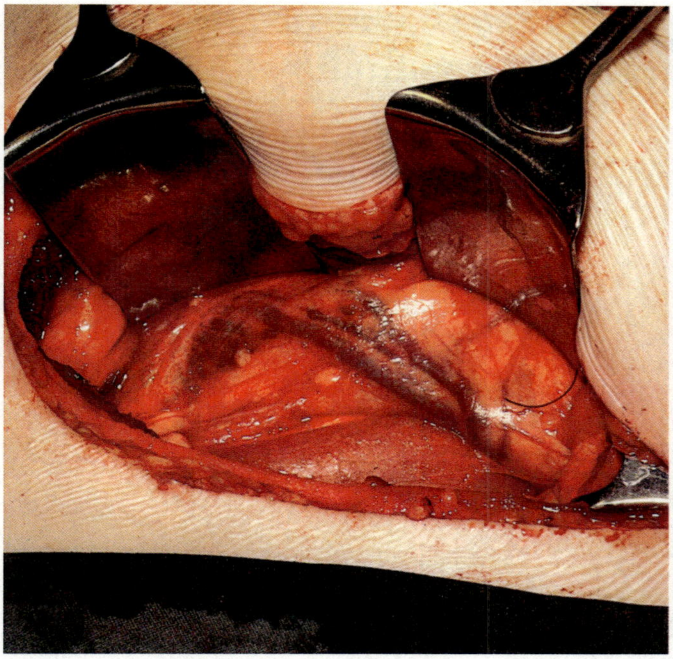

14

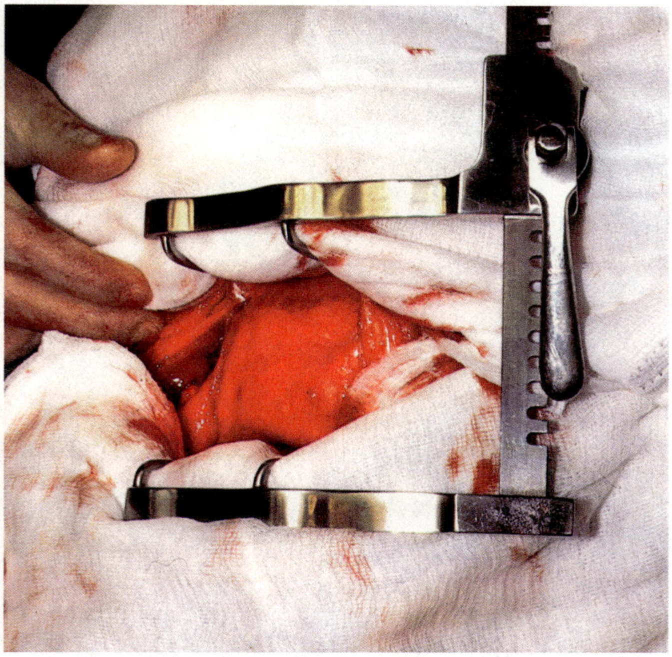

13 The medial side of the psoas is cleaned. (Note the veins attached to the peritoneum, which again can cause severe haemorrhage.) The ureter is now coming into view.

In tuberculous cases, it is easier to feel the ureter before it is seen, because often there is considerable inflammation, and consequently a tendency for venous ooze. This can be controlled by diathermy coagulation or by the application of oxidised cellulose or a similar coagulant.

14 The peritoneum has been reflected, and self-retaining retractor inserted, the edges of the wound being protected by large sways. A good deal of care should be taken not to traumatise and tear the peritoneum.

15

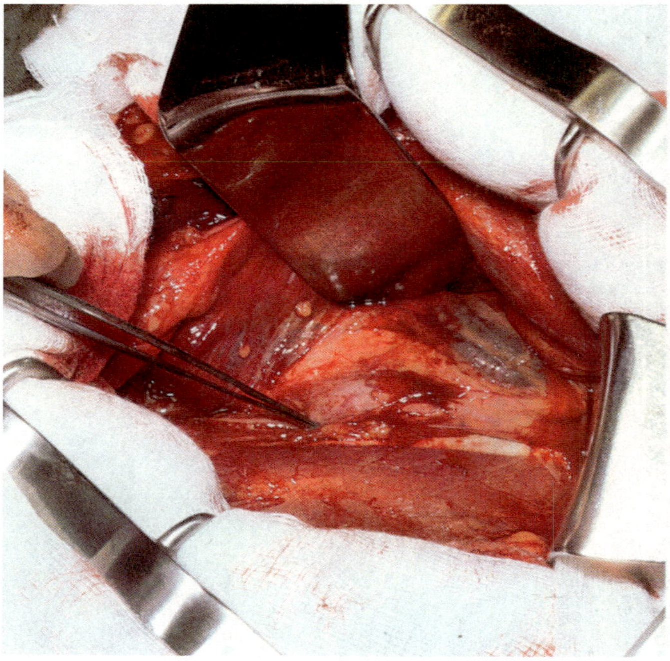

16

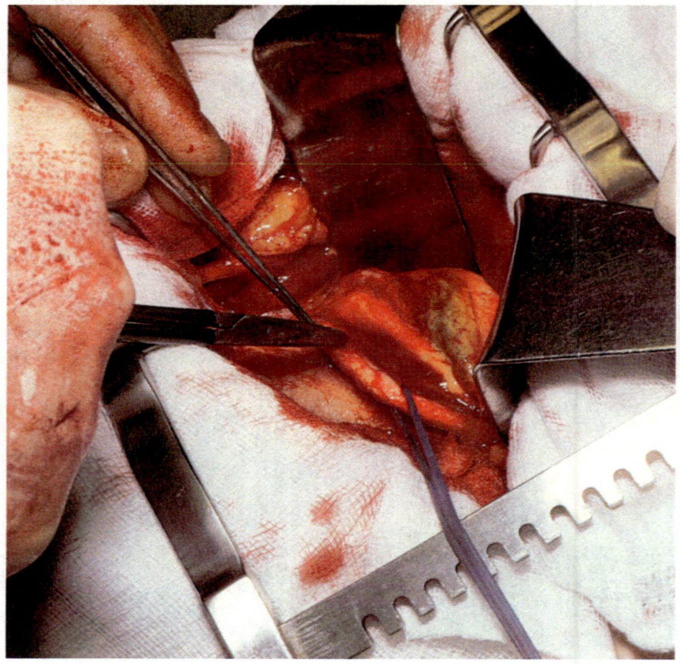

15 The ureter has come into view. It is denoted by the tip of the forceps. The ureter is thickened, rather purply in colour, which is the usual findings with tuberculous infection, and it is inflamed proximal to the purple area.

16 The ureter is dissected carefully until normal ureter is obtained; a sling of thin rubber is placed underneath to elevate the ureter and facilitate easier dissection. The length of diseased ureter will decide the dimensions of the flap, but a defect of up to 16cm can be bridged.

Stage 2

17 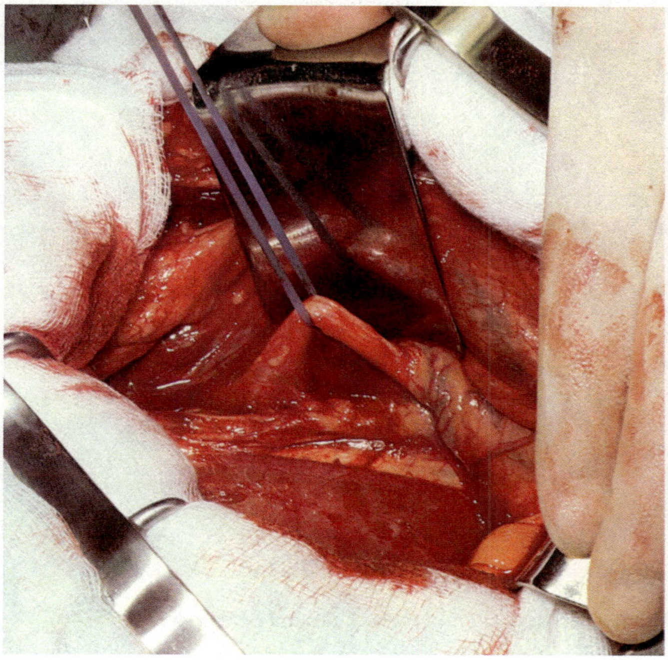

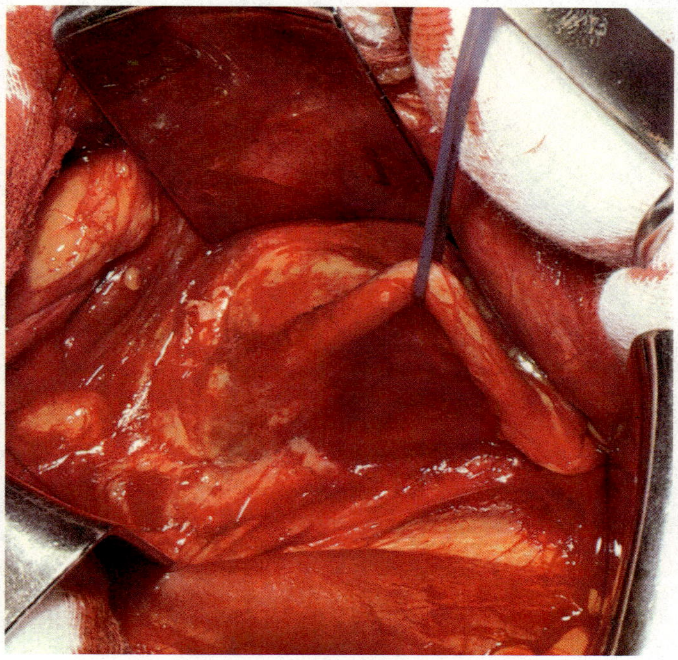 18

17 The ureter is being dissected down towards the bladder. This step may be technically difficult if the ureter is thickened, if peri-ureteric inflammation is present, and if the thickening of the ureter has been present for some time, causing a considerable amount of fibrosis.

There are also some small veins tracking across the ureter just as it enters the bladder. These veins must be coagulated by diathermy as soon as they are seen, to prevent severe haemorrhage. If diathermy fails to control the bleeding, Liga clips are usually successful.

18 The dissected ureter is being elevated, and the junction with the bladder can be clearly seen.

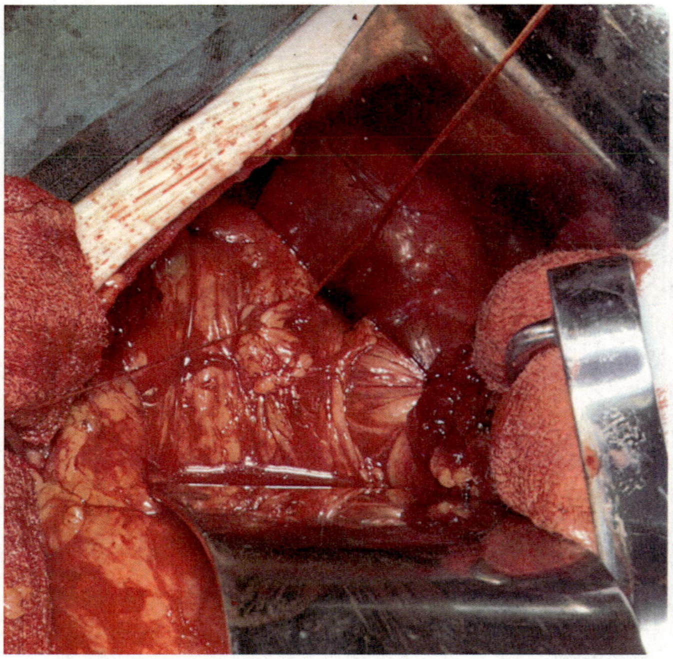

20

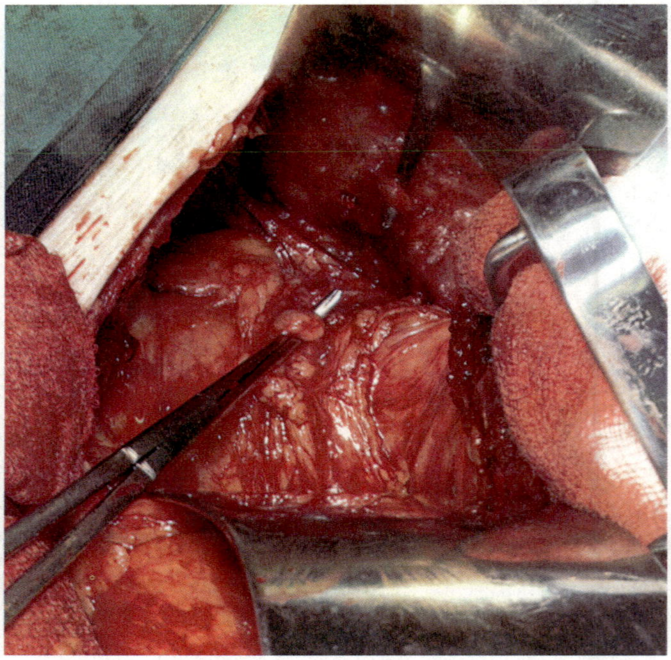

19 The next stage is to mark carefully the base of the flap; two stay sutures are being inserted into the fundus of the bladder. It is important to insert the sutures at this stage of the operation, because the bladder wall is relatively thick and the danger of perforation is minimised.

20 Dissection and isolation of the contralateral right ureter.

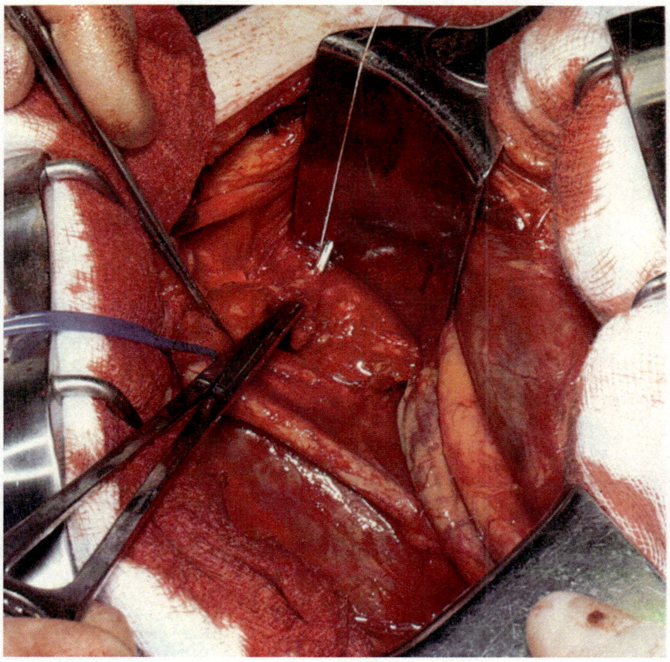

21 **The right superior vesical vessels, which are cut between ligatures to facilitate mobilisation of the bladder.**

22

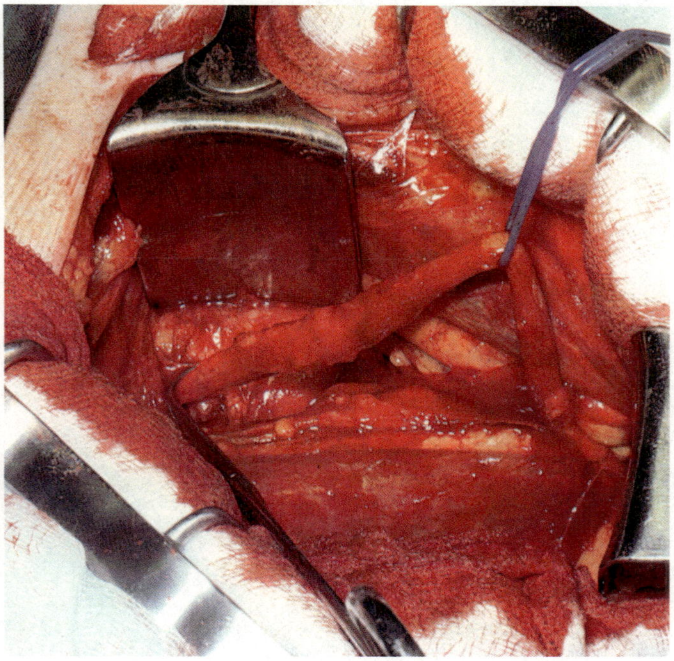

22 **The next stage is to section the left ureter, which is cut close to the bladder, and the vesical end ligated after being transfixed.** Care should be taken not to perforate the numerous small vessels in that area.

23

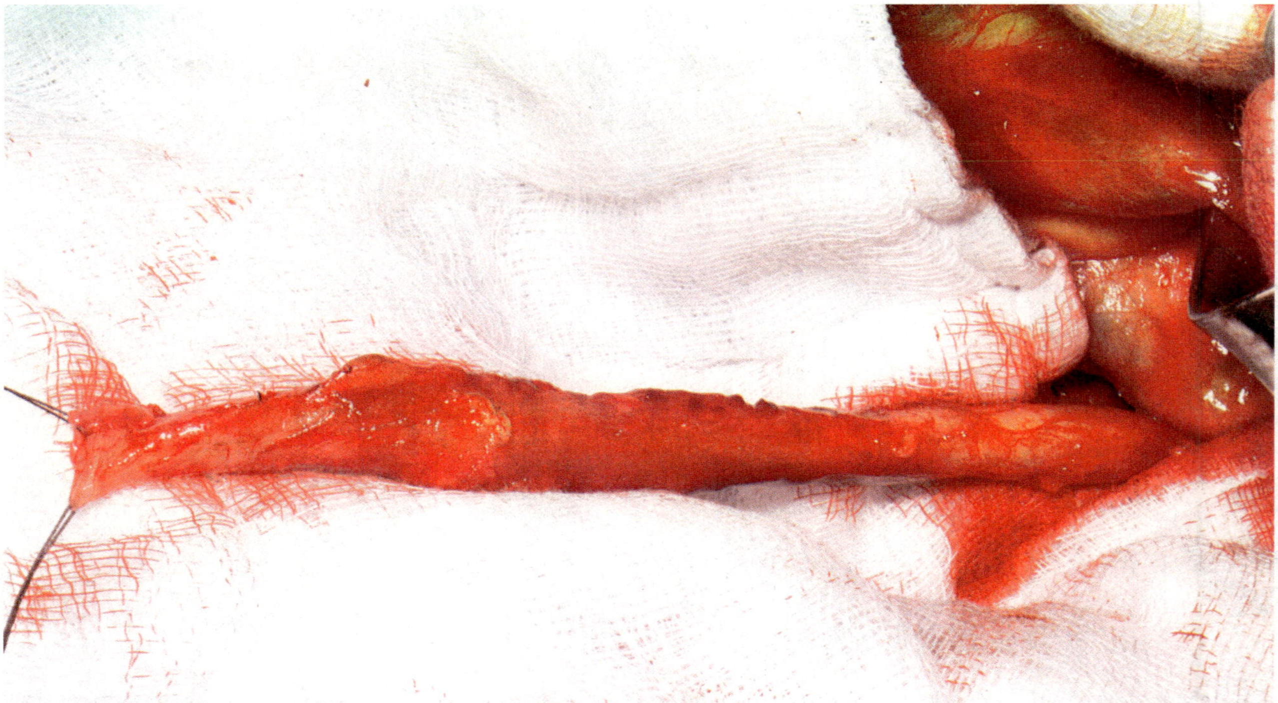

23 The cut ureter is exposed, and is laid on the surface, so that all the diseased tissue can be removed. At least 1cm of normal ureter should be excised with the diseased part to be certain that all damaged tissue is removed.

24 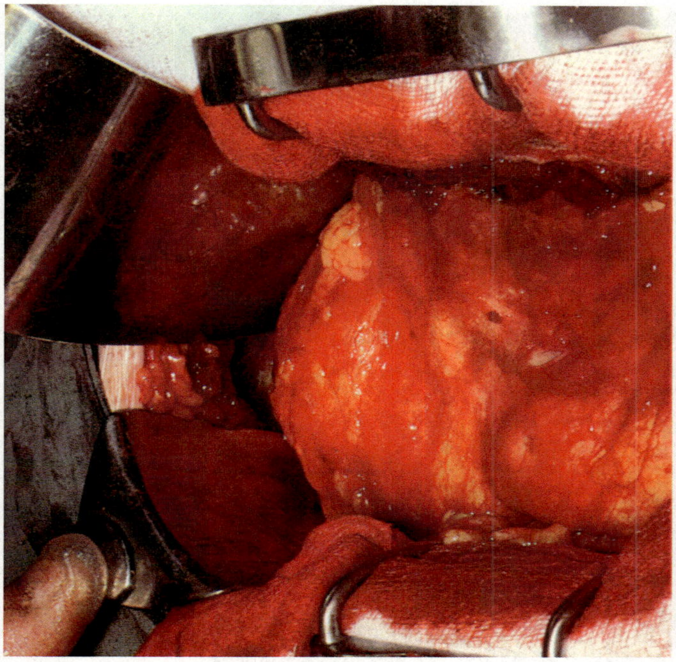

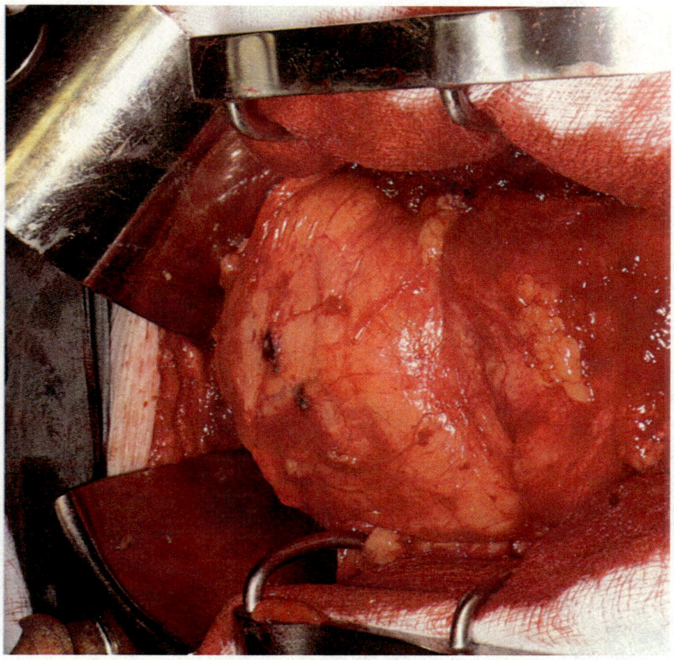 25

24 and 25 The bladder being filled, the reservoir connected to the catheter has been opened. When the bladder contains between 200 and 300ml the reservoir is closed, and the peritoneum dissected from the fundus of the bladder.

26

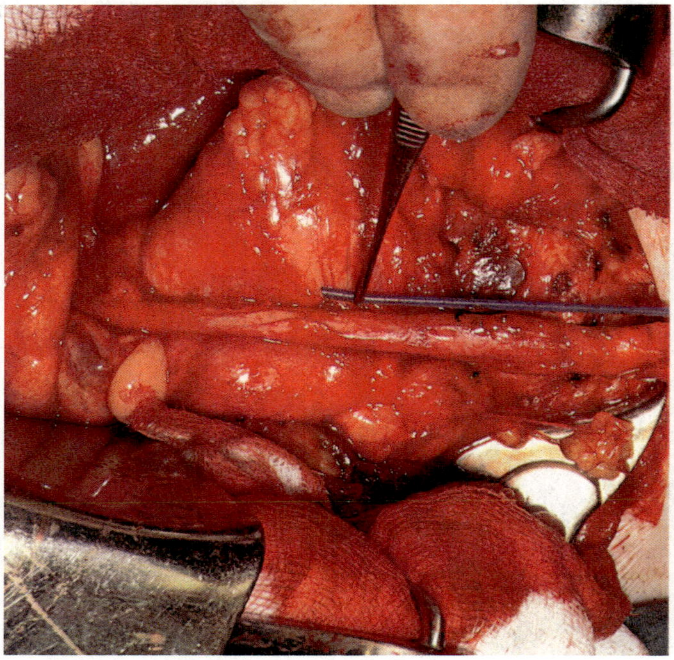

27

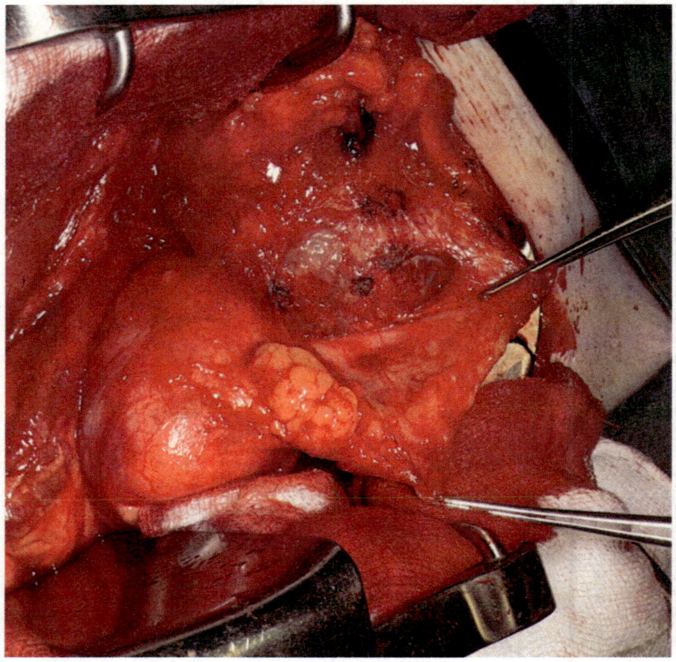

26 The small vessels which communicate with the bladder and peritoneum are coagulated with diathermy.

27 The cut ureter is then placed on the fundus of the bladder, and the length of ureter to be sectioned is measured carefully, by using the thin rubber strip. The two stay sutures are then elevated and the base of the flap is cut.

28 After the bladder is distended to this extent, the wall is extremely thin. Therefore it is important to place the stay sutures at the early stages of the procedure, when the bladder is flaccid.

28

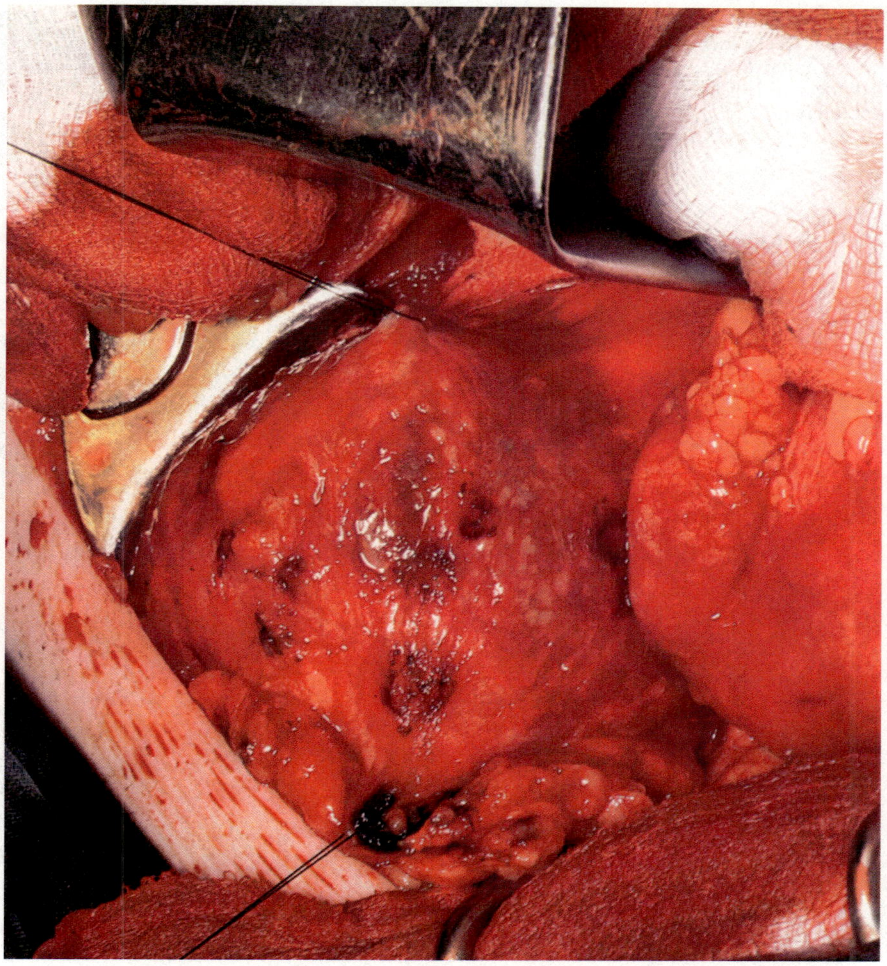

29 The bladder is then dissected free, especially the right hand side, so that the flap can be cut accurately.

29

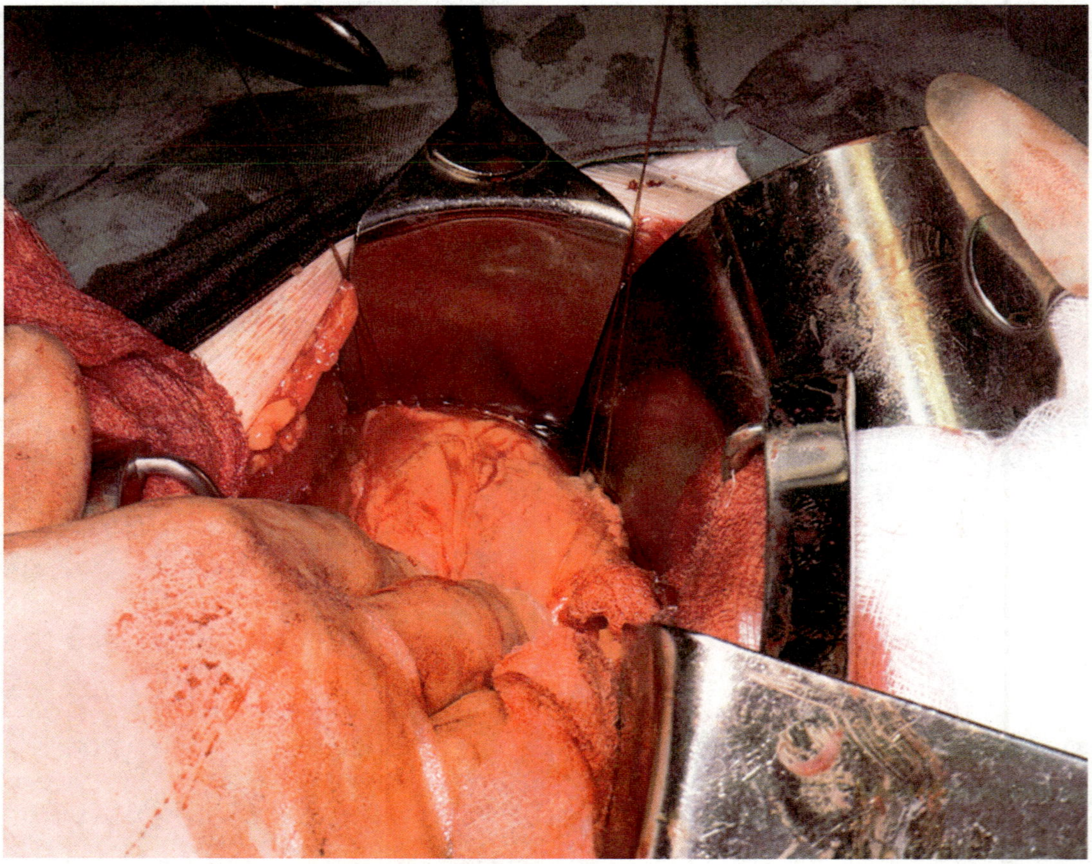

30

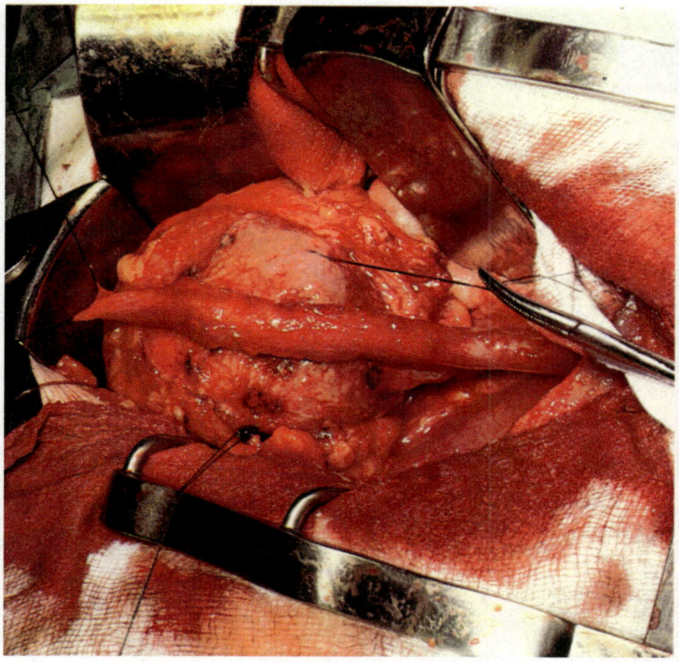

31

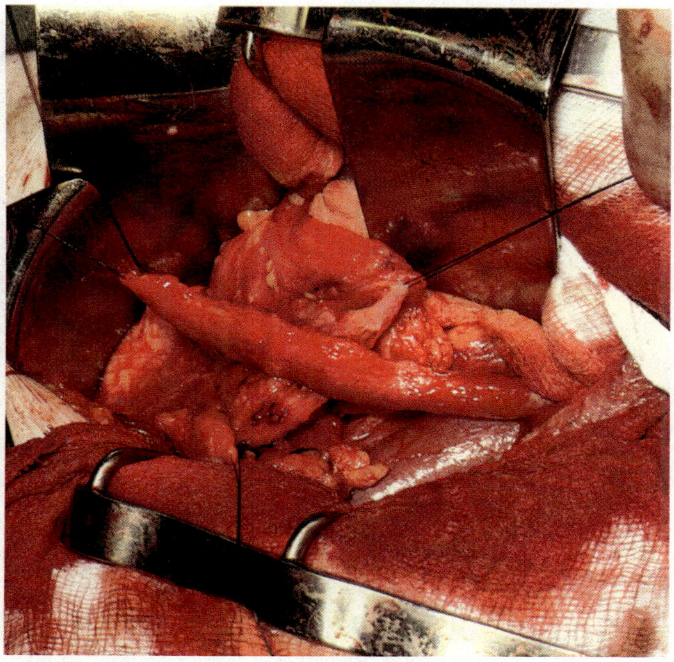

30 and 31 The ureter, which has had the diseased area removed, is then placed over the bladder, so that the length of the flap can be precisely measured with a ruler. When measuring the flap, it is important to ensure that the sub-mucous tunnel will be at least 5 cm in length.

32 The bladder is then opened using fine scissors, with the measured flap prepared.

32

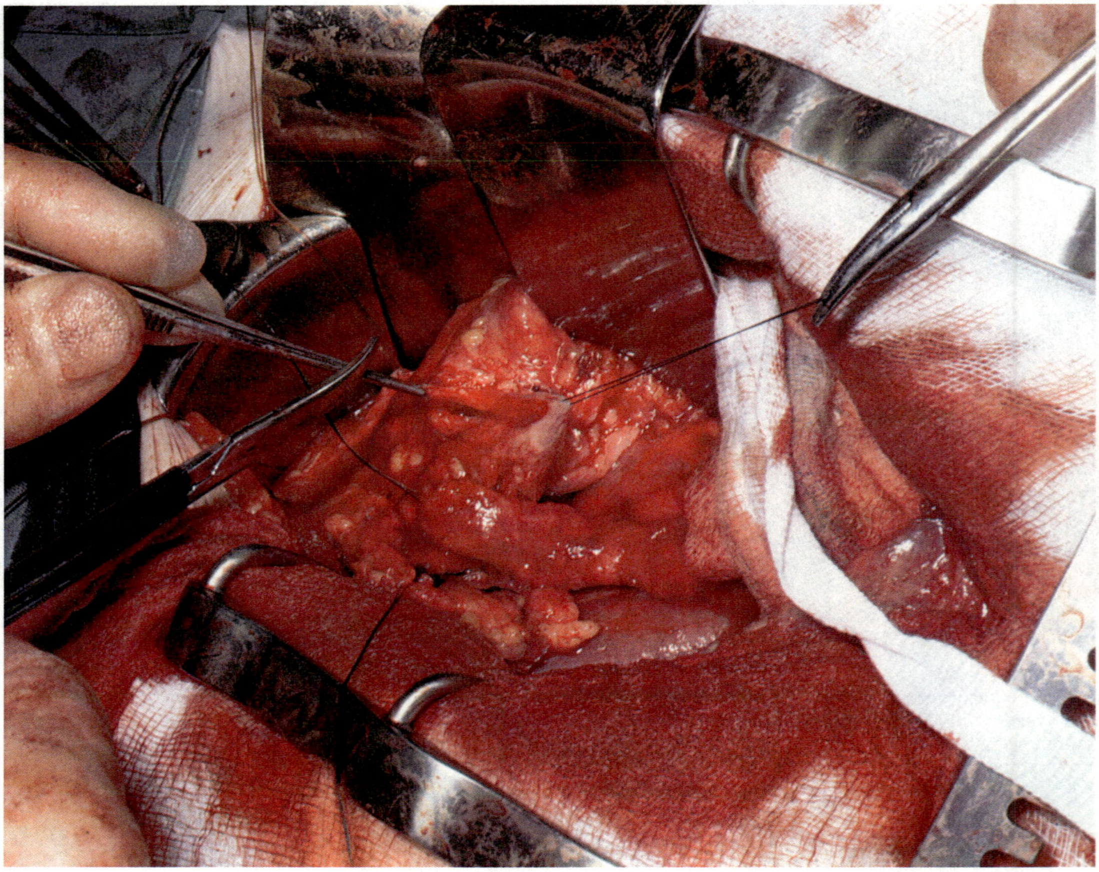

33 At this stage, the contralateral right ureteric orifice is identified and catheterised with a large catheter. The catheter used is about size 6, and is placed up the ureter so that the ureter can be felt easily if it is necessary to continue the flap over the right side of the bladder. This procedure should be performed carefully because it is possible to perforate the ureter. This precaution is not often necessary, because it is rare for the length of the flap to reach over the far side of the bladder so that it is in close proximity to the opposite ureteric orifice.

33

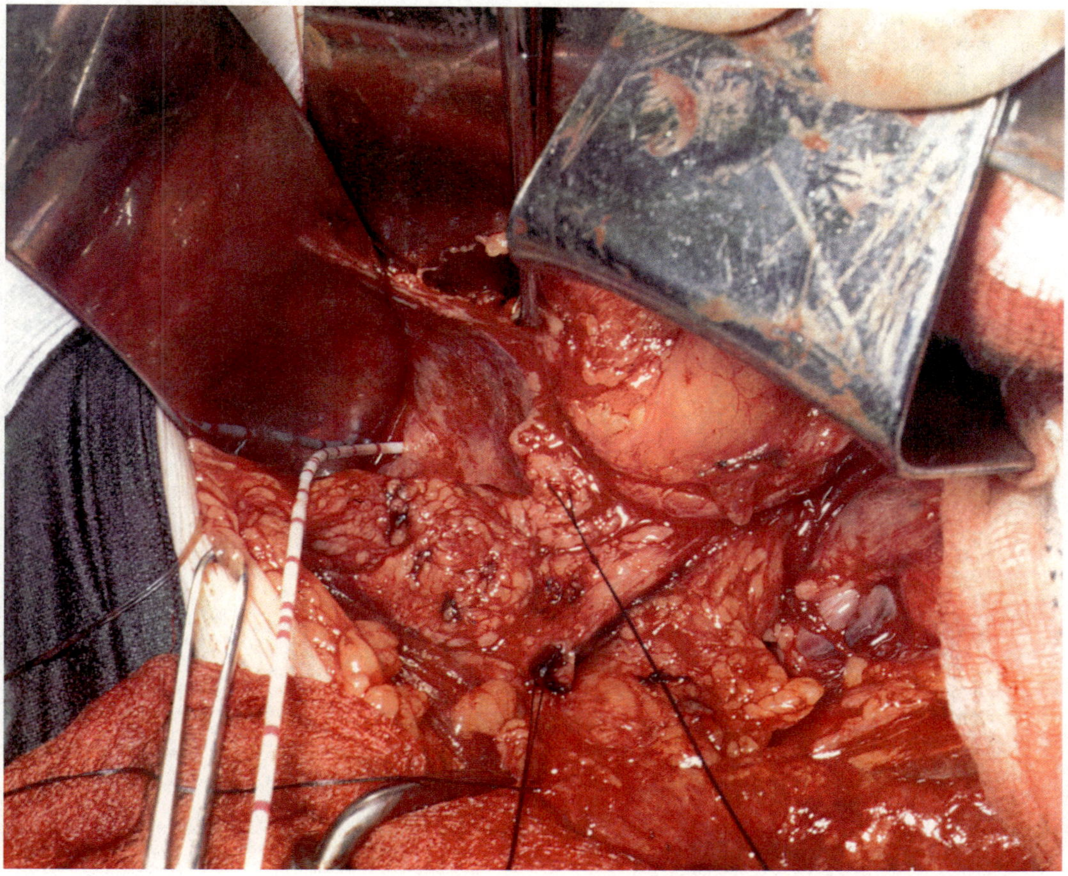

34 The flap with a broad base. Note that because of the good blood supply to the bladder, the width of the flap is much narrower than would be expected for a normal skin flap.

34

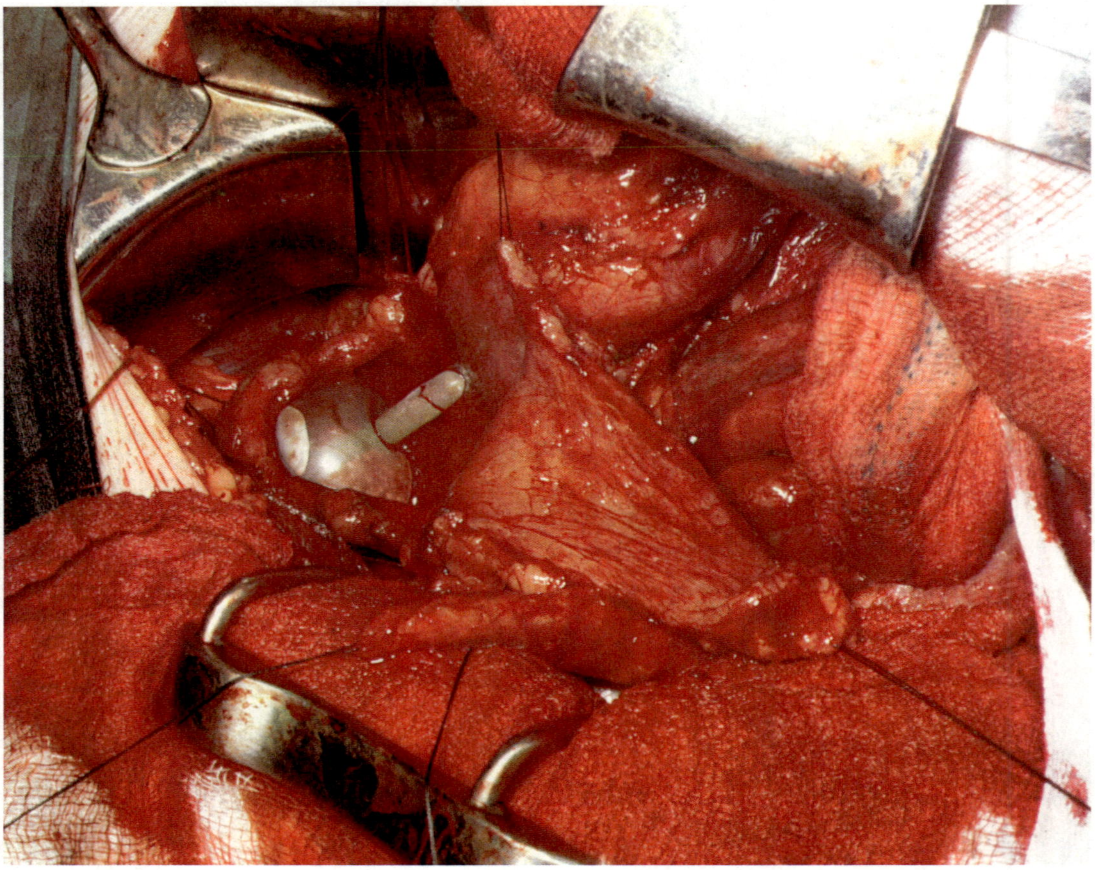

35

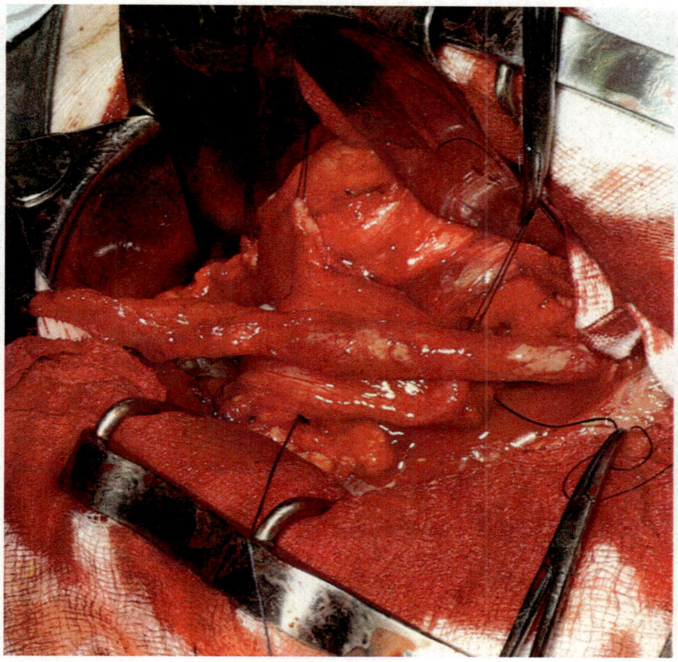

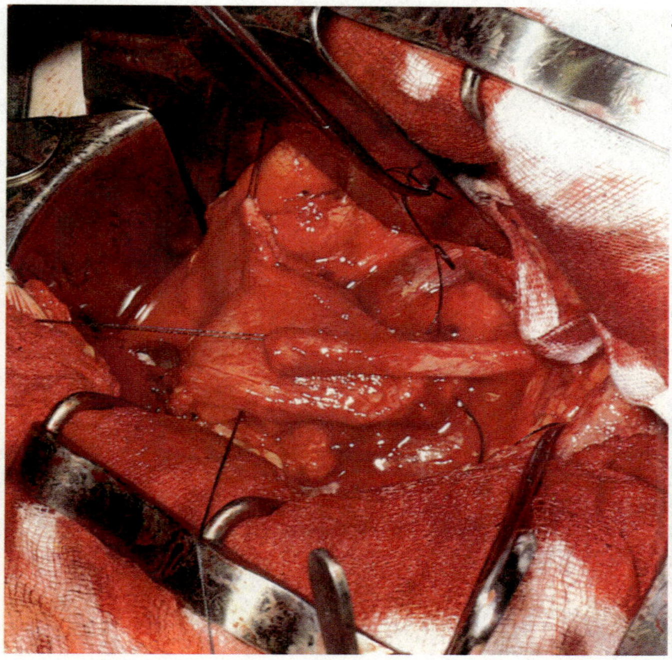

36

35 The ureter is placed over the flap.

36 The redundant ureter is excised. Note the stay suture at the end of the ureter, which is of invaluable assistance when the ureter is being introduced into the tunnel. The suture is inserted after the redundant ureter has been excised.

37

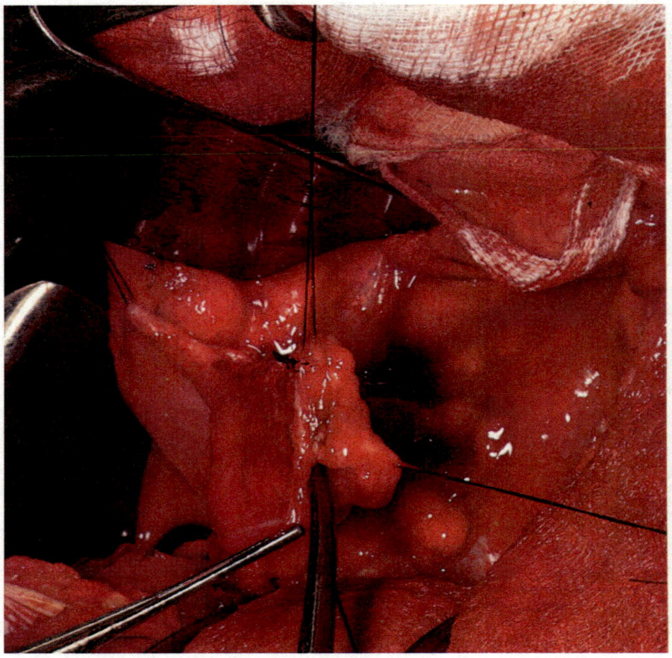

38

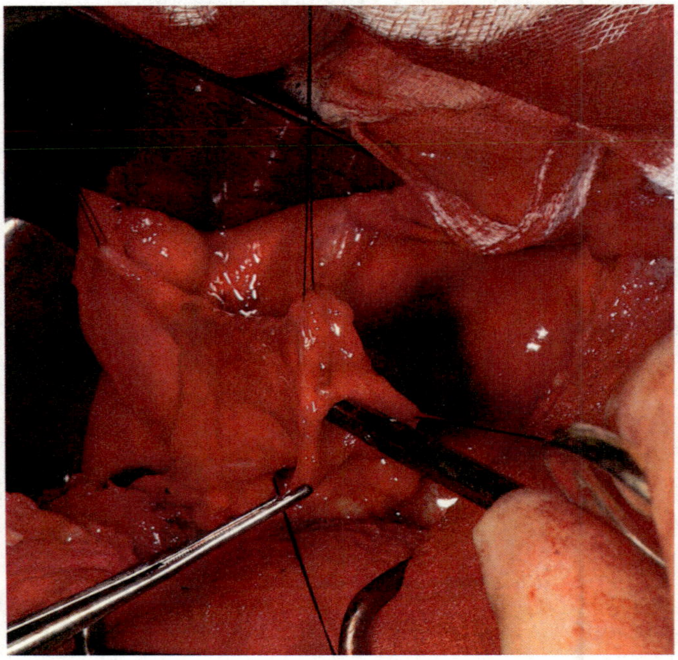

37 and 38 The sub-mucous tunnel is being prepared, using fine blunt-pointed scissors. It is important to try and keep as close to the mucous membrane as possible, otherwise it may be very difficult to thread the ureter through the tunnel. The plane between the bladder mucous membrane and the muscle is ideal. Either curved scissors, or scissors which are angled on the flat, are the best instruments for this particular part of the operation. The scissors may be seen underneath the mucous membrane, approaching the base of the flap.

39 A further view of the tip of the scissors about to come through the mucous membrane. Note the 5cm satisfactory length of the tunnel.

39

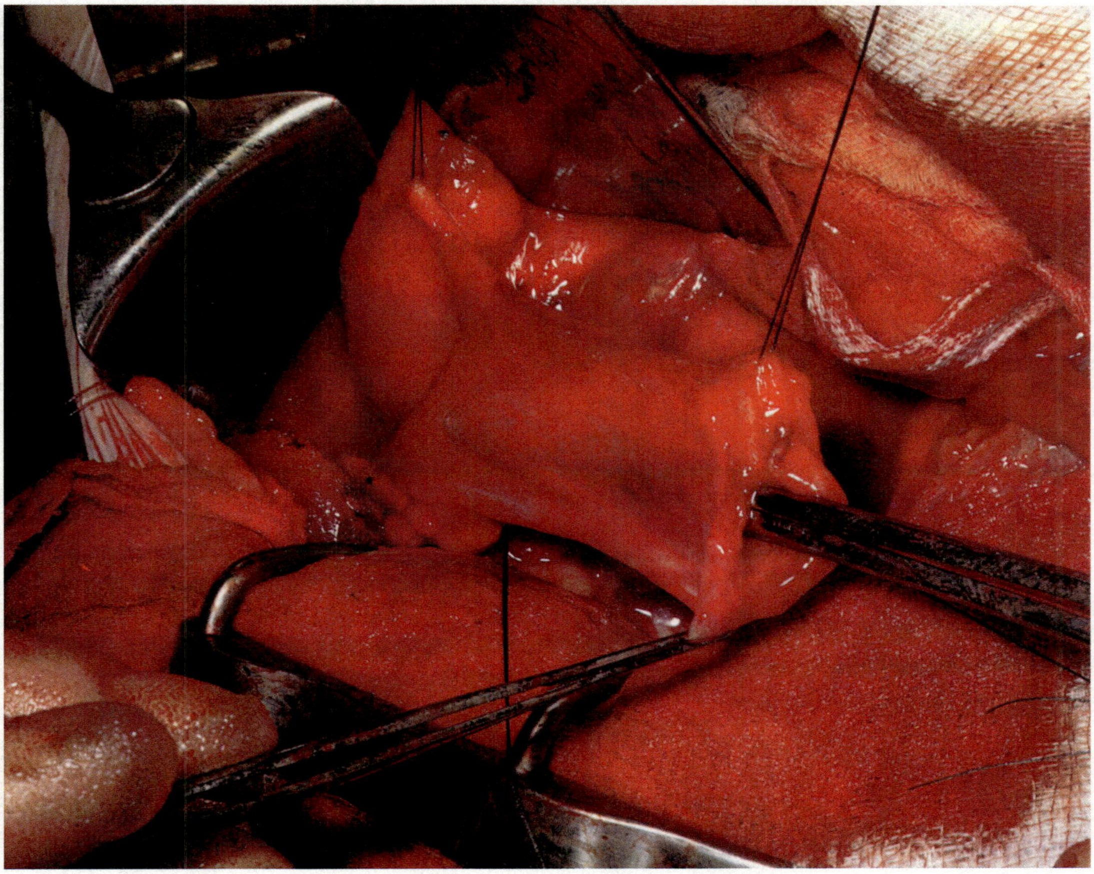

40 Before the ureter is threaded through the tunnel, it is spatulated to facilitate anastomosis of the ureter to the mucous membrane. The spatulation should be planned carefully to prevent rotation of the ureter after it has been threaded through the tunnel into the bladder. At this stage, some urologists form a cuff at the lower end of the ureter. However, I do not think this is necessary, and only adds to the duration of the operative procedure. Provided that one gets adequate tunnel, there is no additional advantage in creating a nipple.

40

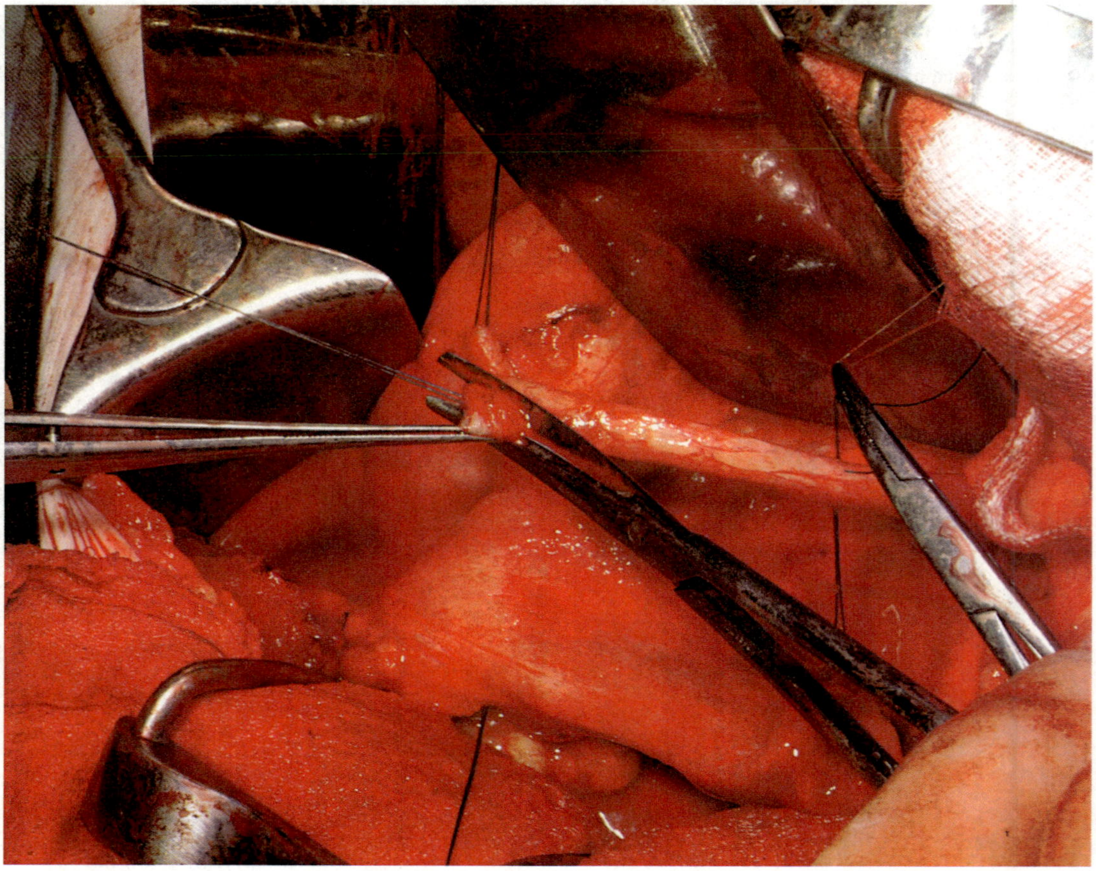

41 The spatulated ureter, which has been held open by skin hooks, which are invaluable instruments at this stage.

41

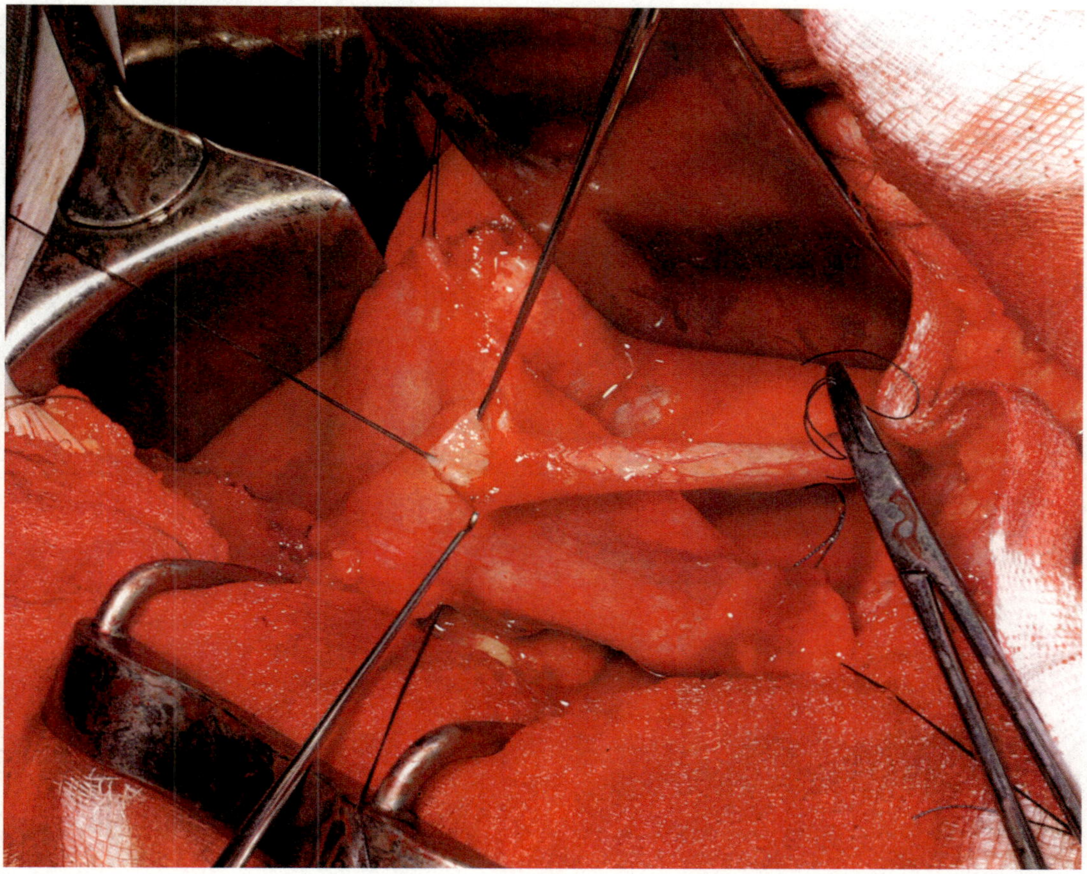

42 The ureter is being threaded gently through the tunnel, using the stay suture for gentle traction. If the ureter does not pass easily into the bladder, the tunnel should be widened.

42

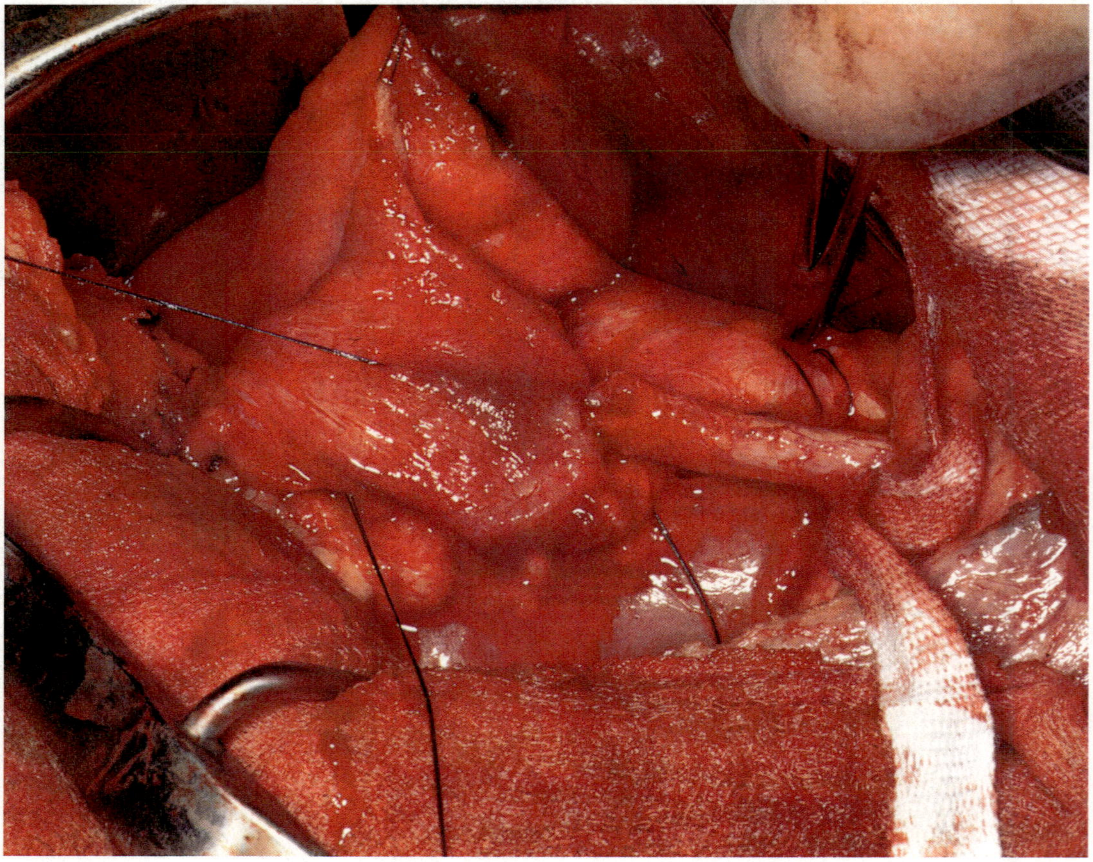

Stage 3

43 The ureter has now been threaded through the tunnel into the bladder and the spatulated end can be seen clearly at the base of the flap.

43

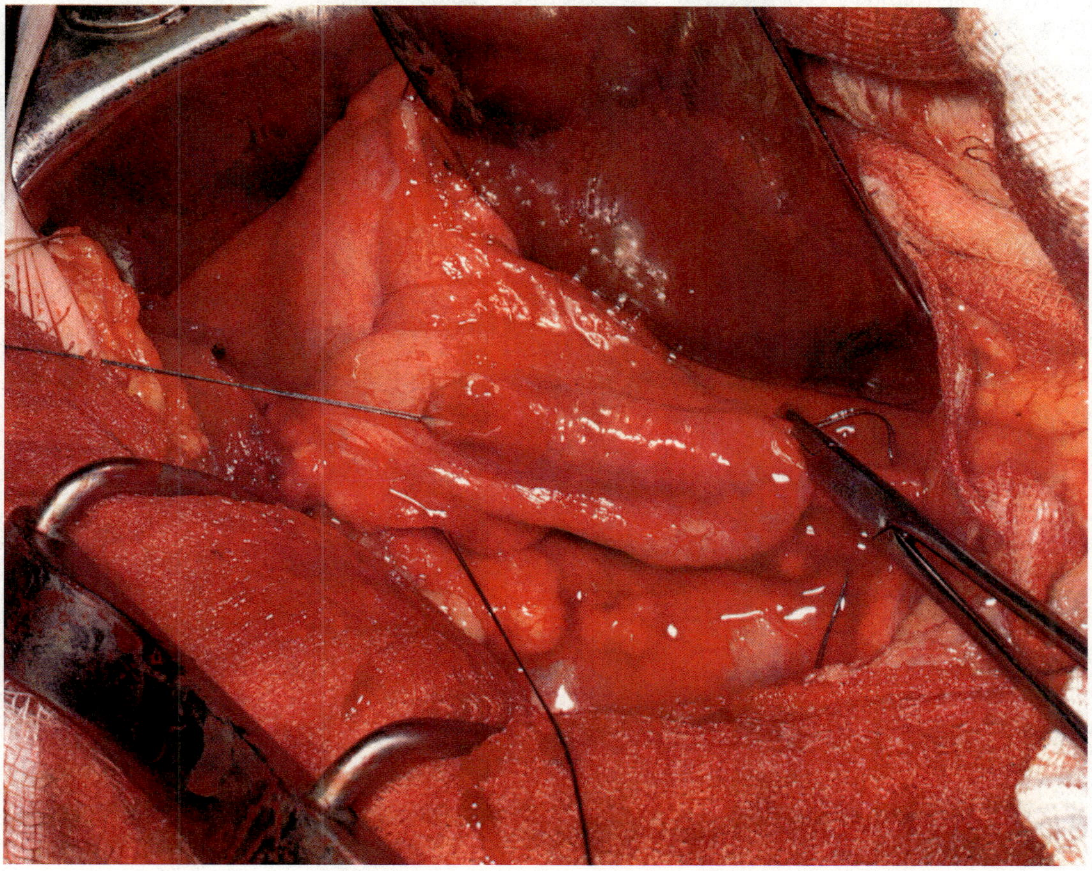

44 The ureter is being sutured to the flap. 4.0 or 5.0 Dexon sutures are used. It is important to ensure that, although a mucosa to mucosa anastomosis is mandatory, a good bite of the bladder muscle is included in the stitch.

44

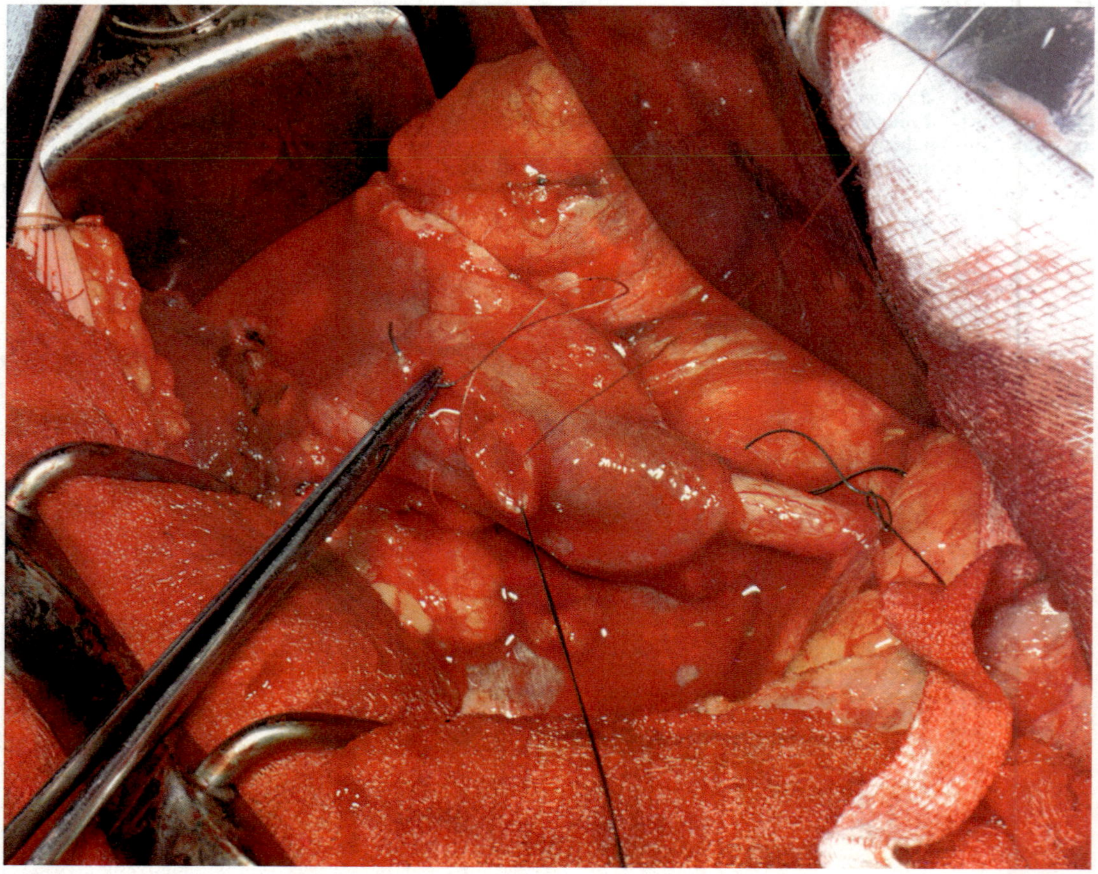

45

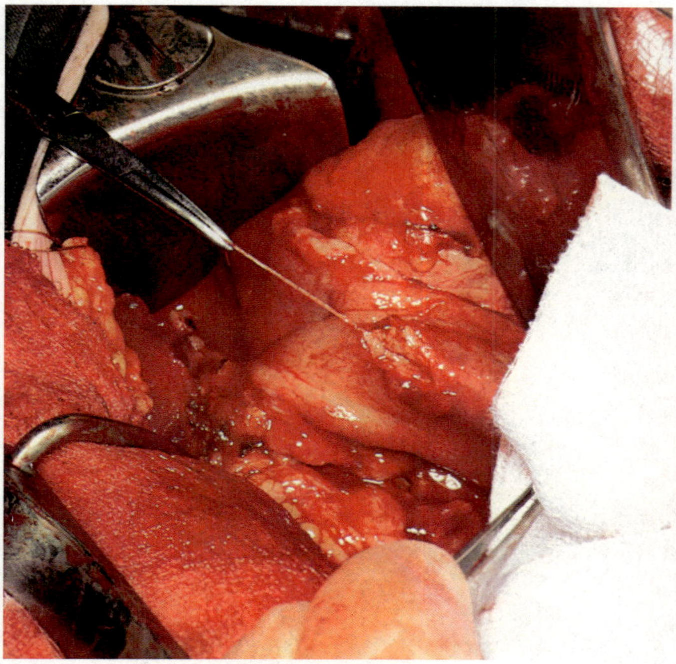

46

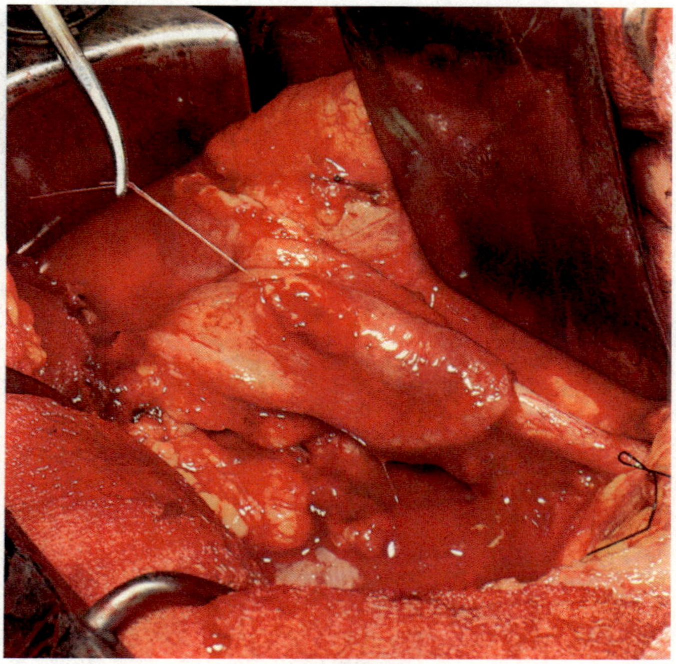

45 and 46 The ureter is situated neatly in the base of the flap. Haemorrhage from the bladder flap can be troublesome, although it is rarely severe. Care should be taken to have small vessels under run when the bladder is being cut, or coagulate them by diathermy.

47 A stent is being introduced into the ureter. The stent is a safety device used when suturing the ureter to the mucous membrane and muscle of the bladder flap.

Some surgeons prefer to leave a stent in the ureter. However, I do not accept this technique because there is evidence, provided by Cukier and Thompson, that the results are better if stents are not used. Also in my series there has been no evidence to suggest that the use of a stent would improve results.

47

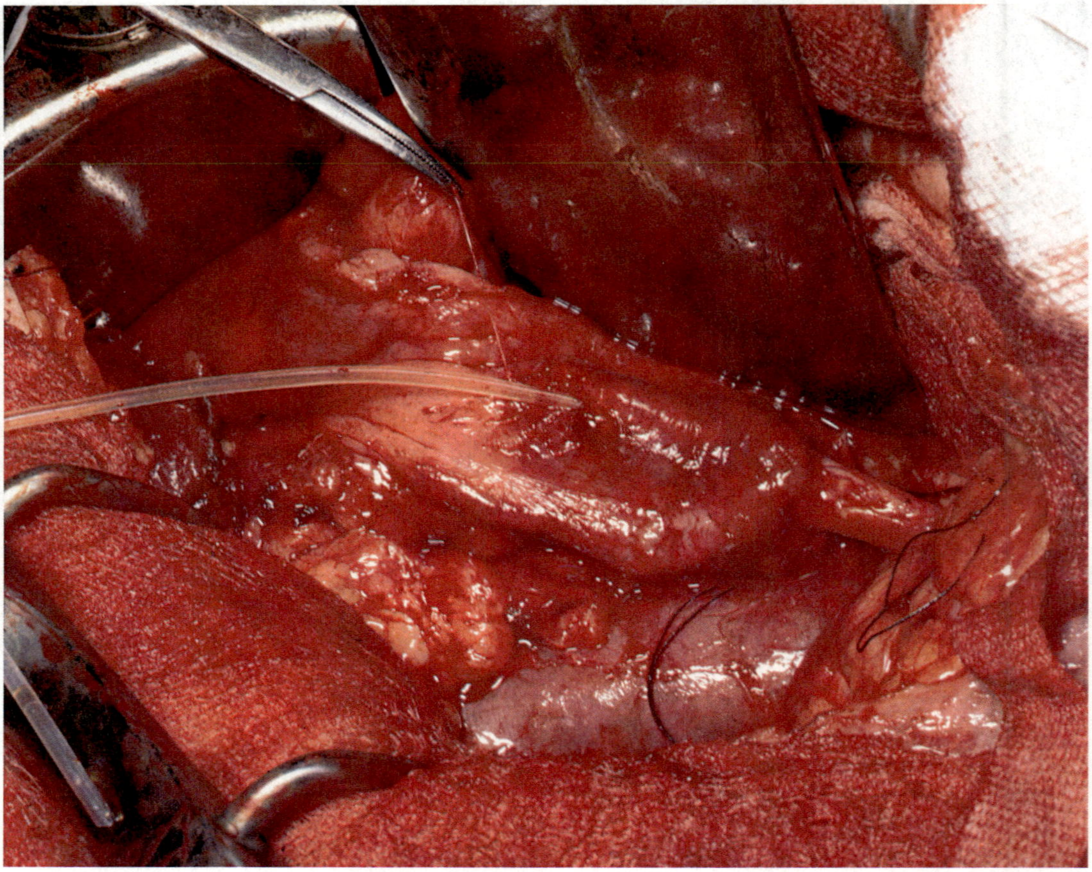

48 Anastomosis has been completed between the spatulated ureter and the bladder flap. There has been a small haematoma under the flap. This is occasionally seen, but does not appear to be of significance, because its presence does not seem to prejudice results.

48

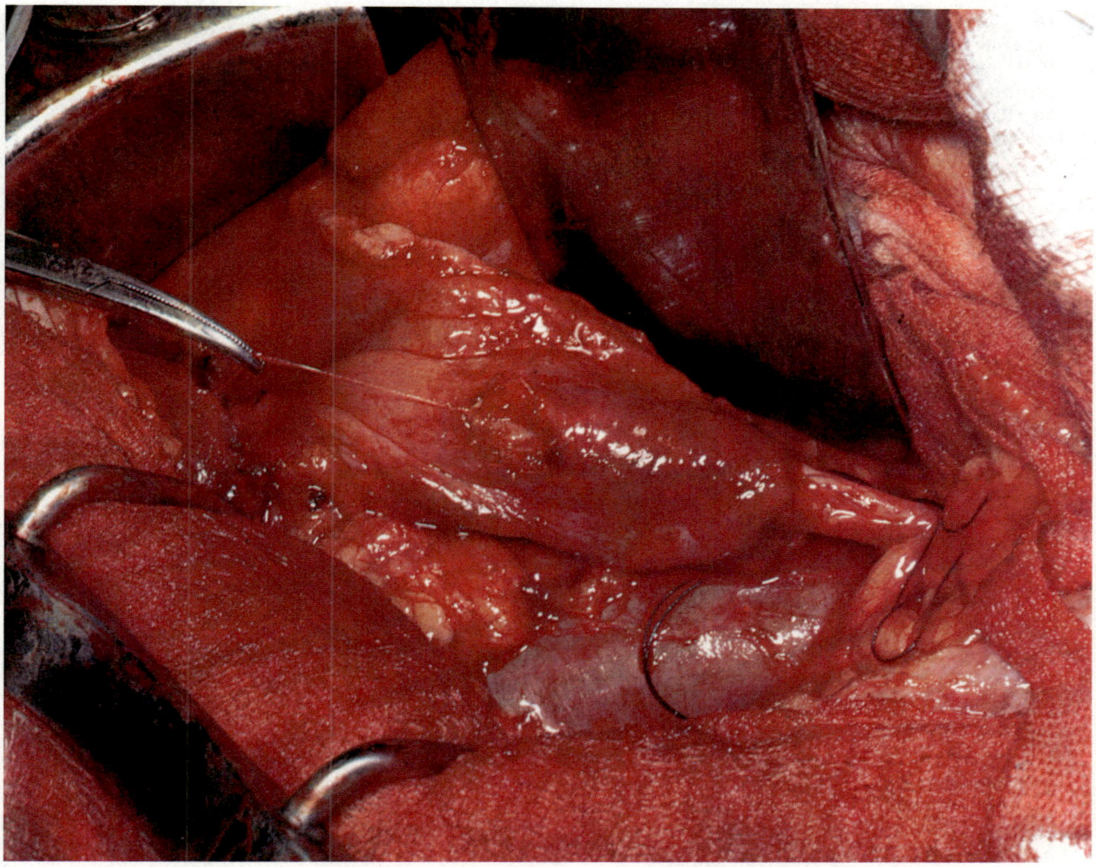

49 The first stitch, which is a fine suture, 4.0 or 5.0 Dexon, has been inserted into the muscle of the flap and the ureter. Three sutures are placed in this position. These are the initial fixation sutures, which help to anchor the flap to the ureter.

49

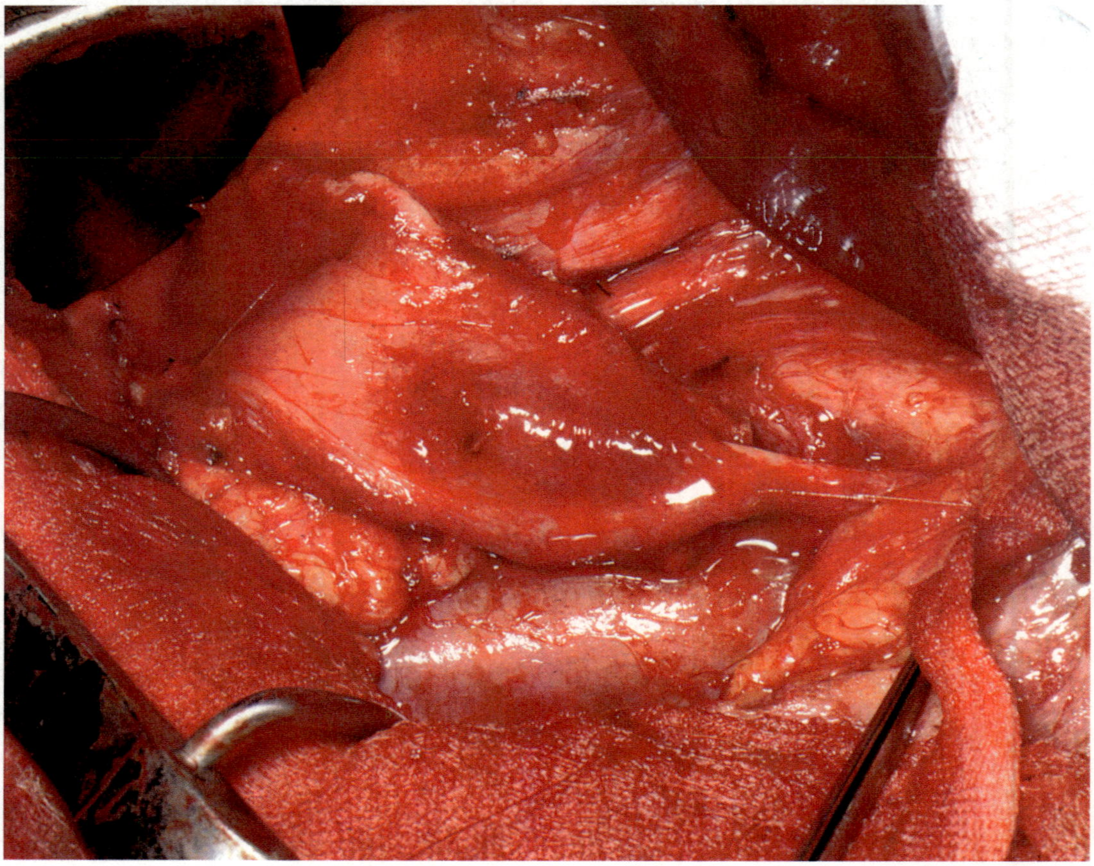

50

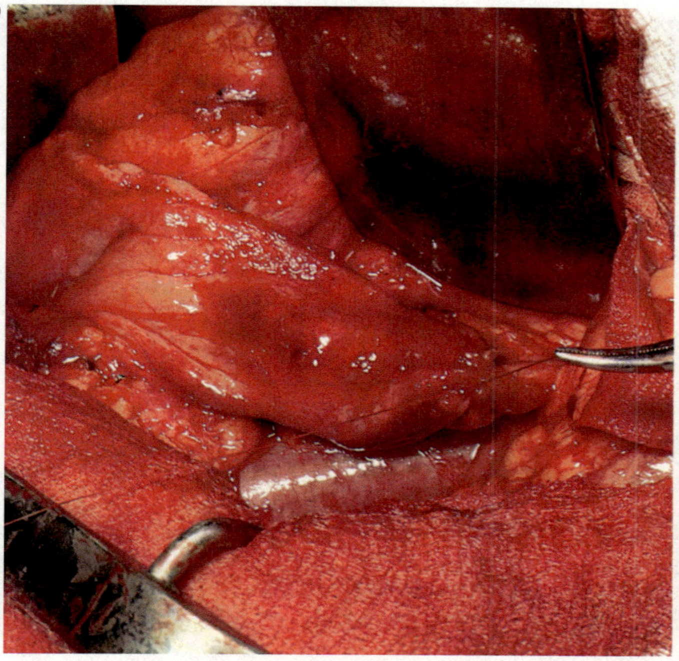

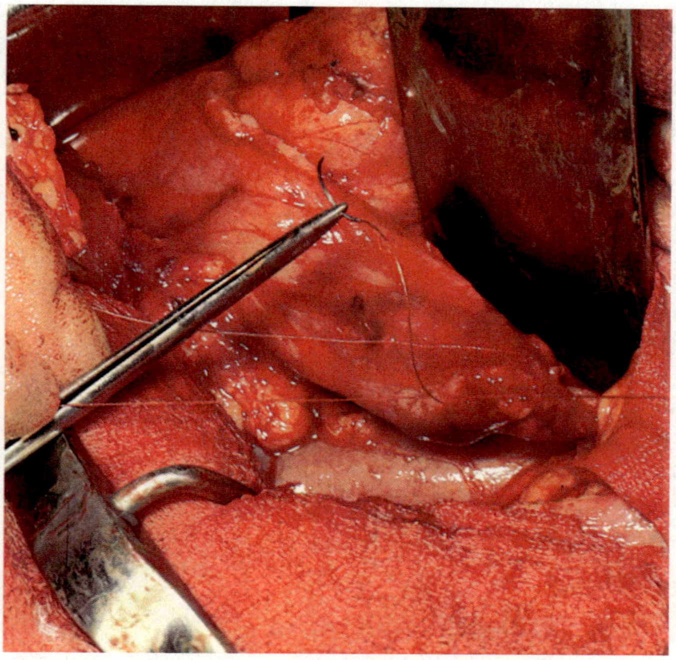

51

50 The closure of the flap. This is carried out with 3.0 Dexon in a two-layer closure.

The first layer is a continuous interlocking suture, the sutures being placed about 2 mm apart. There are many equally satisfactory methods of suturing, but the choice must be the surgeon's.

51 The start of the suture at the apex of the flap.

53

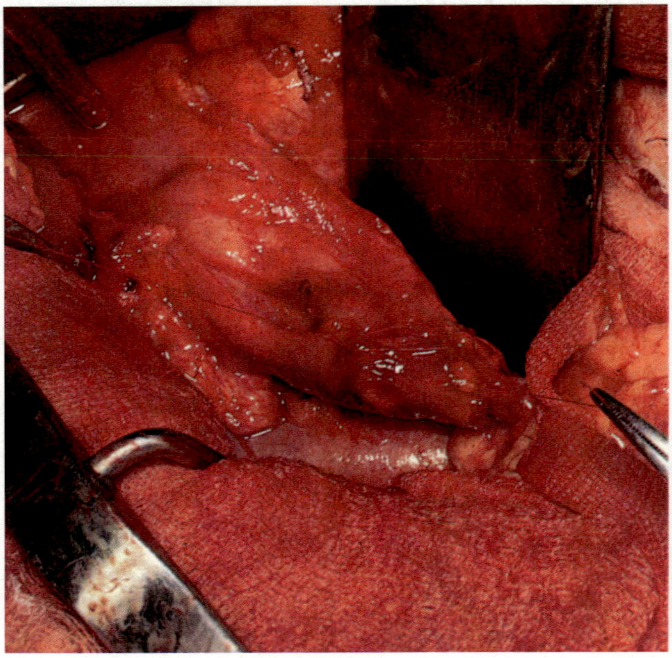

52

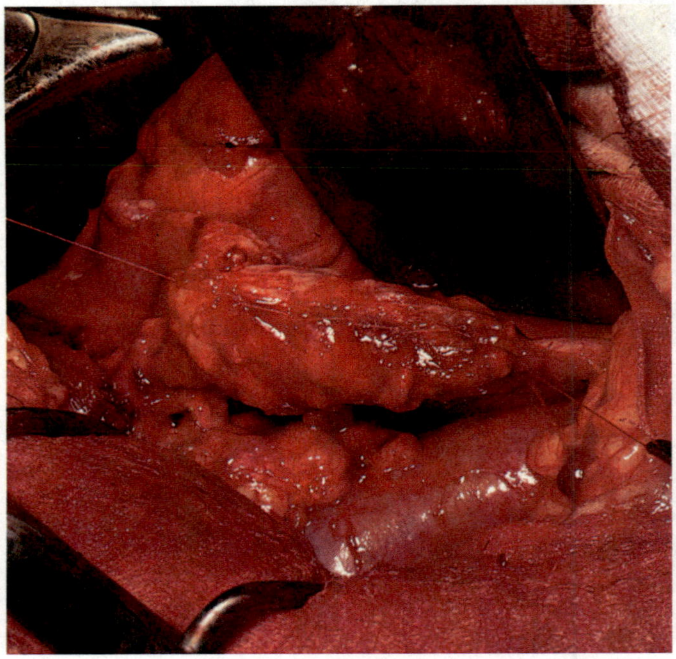

52 The flap half closed.

53 The flap completely closed and the suture continuing to close the bladder.

54 **This stitch is carried out right through to the base of the bladder**; the balloon of the Foley catheter can be seen clearly.

54

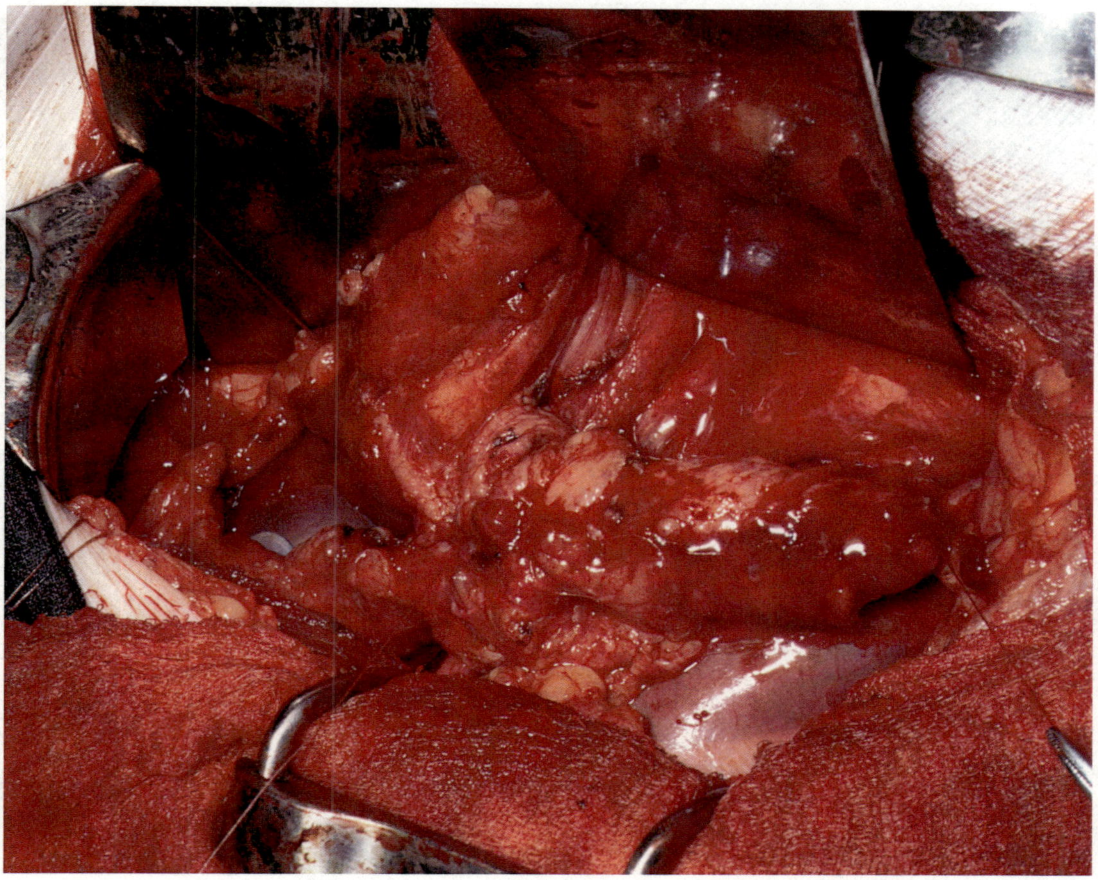

55 Closure of the first layer has been completed.

55

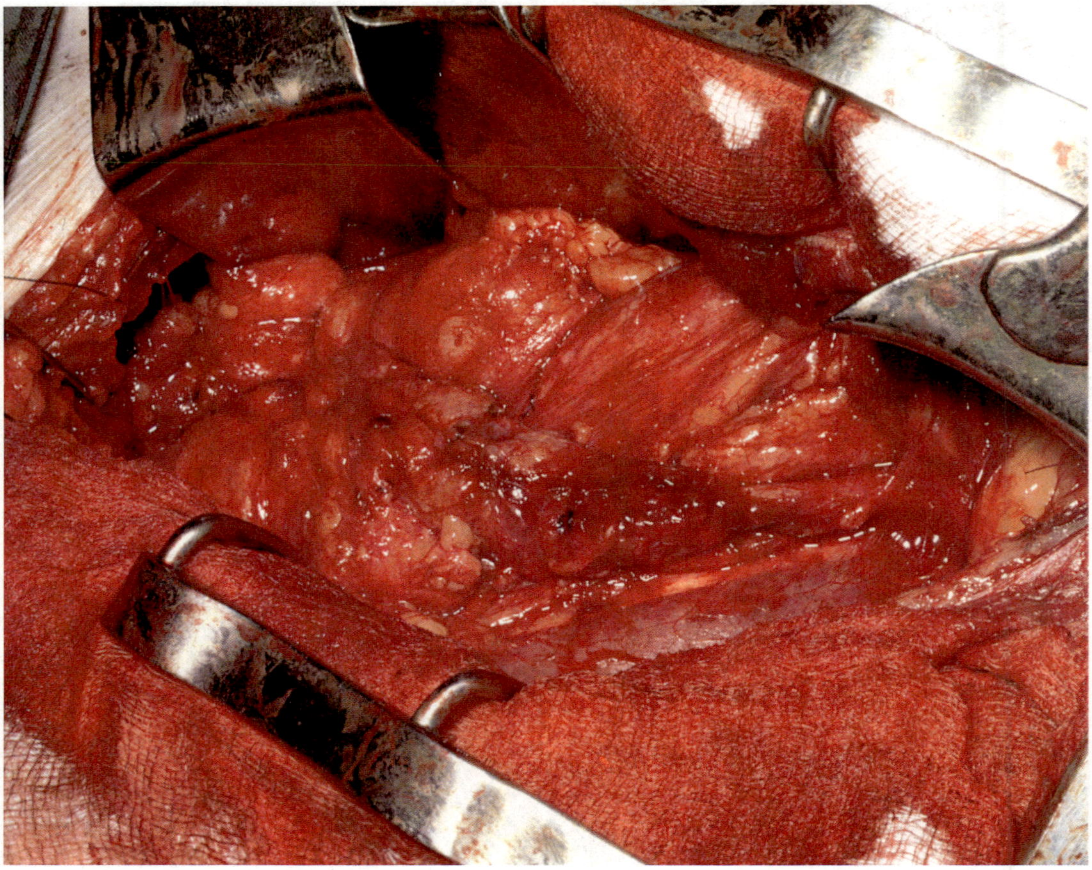

56

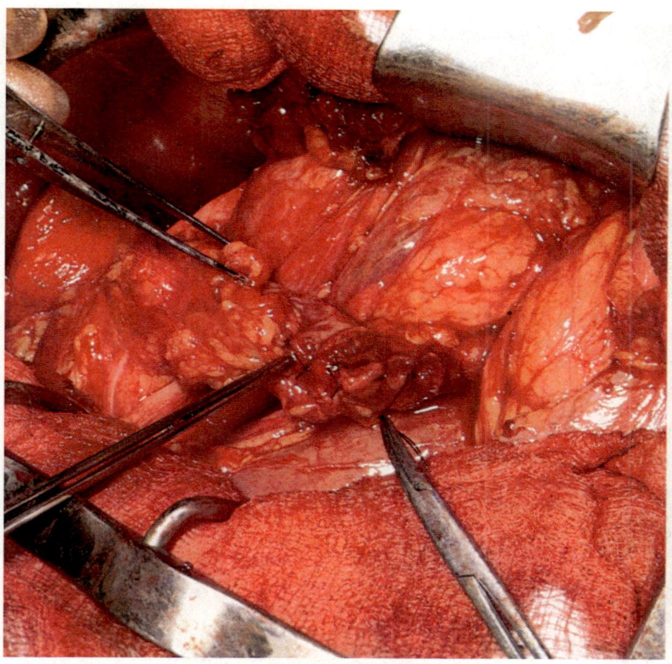

57

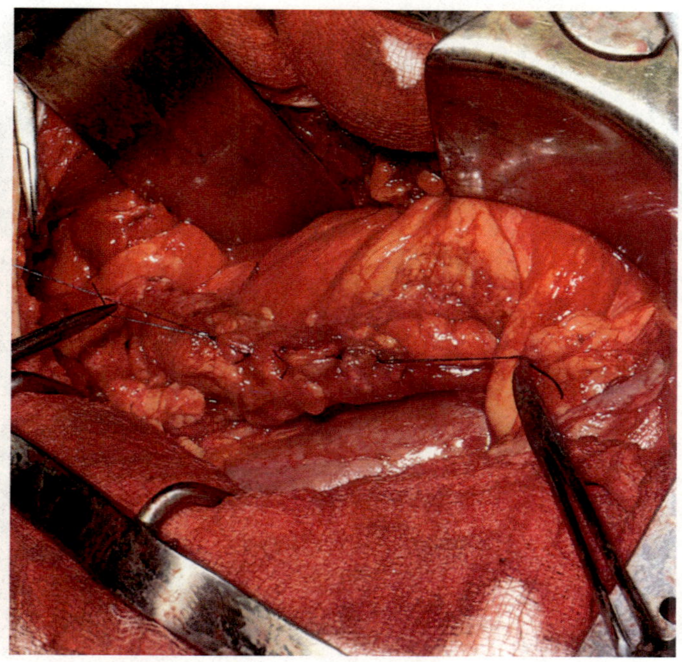

56 and 57 The second layer is again closed by using 3.0 Dexon with a continuous running stitch, starting at the base of the bladder.

58 The final sutures, which are interrupted Dexon, either 4.0 or 5.0, have been inserted between the muscle of the ureter and the apex of the bladder flap. These sutures are placed about 3 mm apart, and are continued through the entire circumference of the ureter.

58

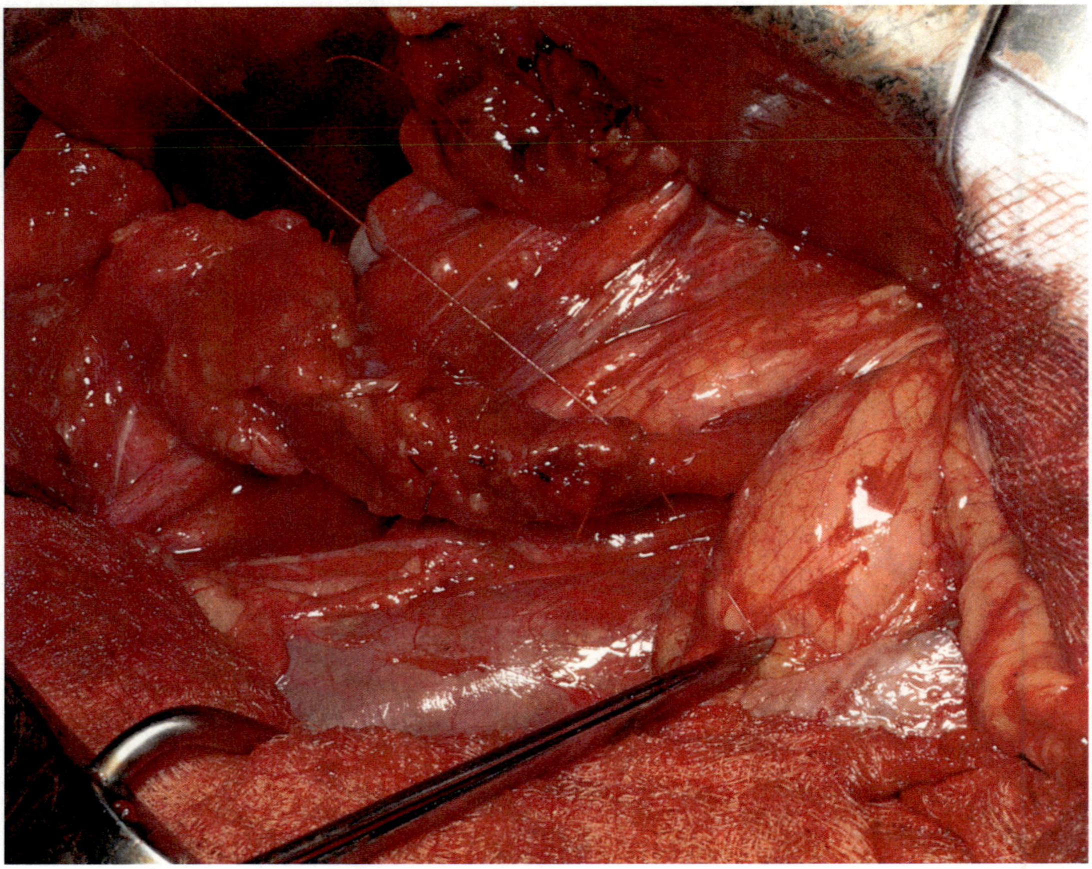

59 **Anastomosis completed**. At this stage the bladder is refilled from the reservoir with 250 ml of saline, so that any leaks can be identified and closed.

59

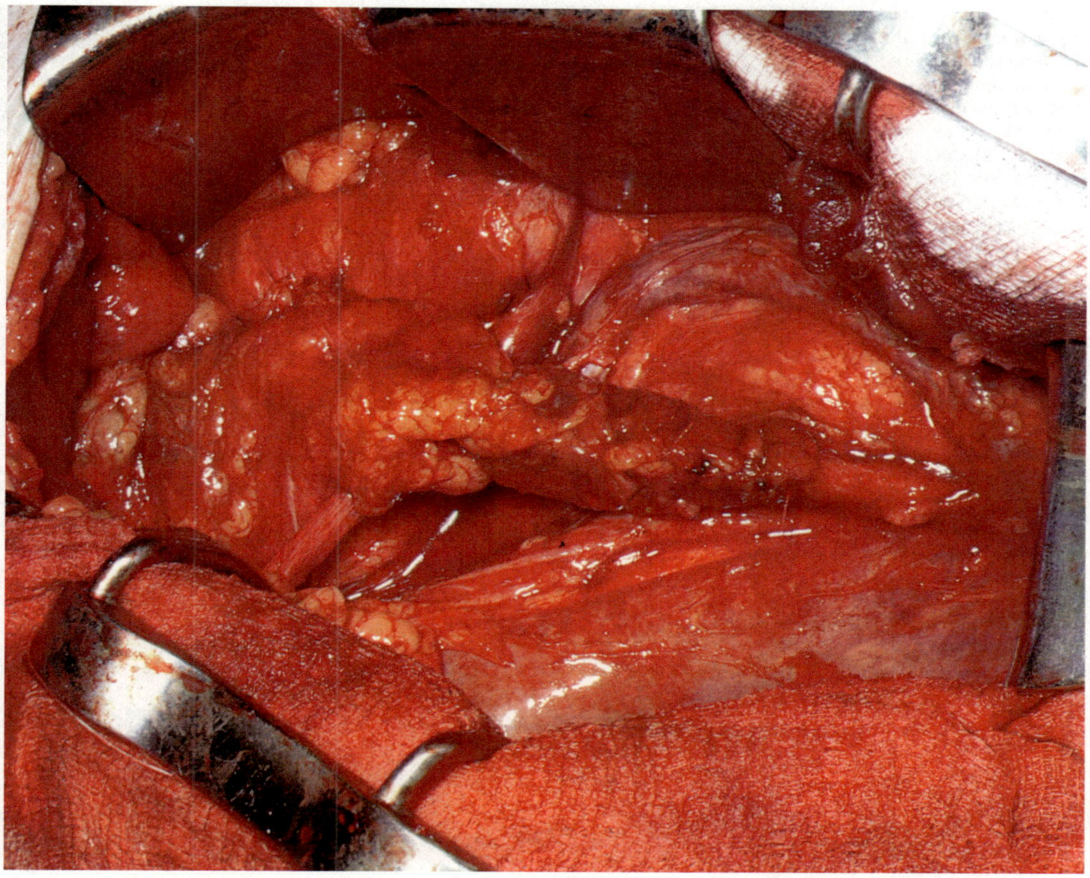

60 The bladder flap being sutured to the psoas muscle. Three or four sutures, using 3.0 Dexon, are used. This is to prevent undue mobility of the bladder flap after the anastomosis, which could possibly prejudice the anastomosis or promote a urinary leak.

60

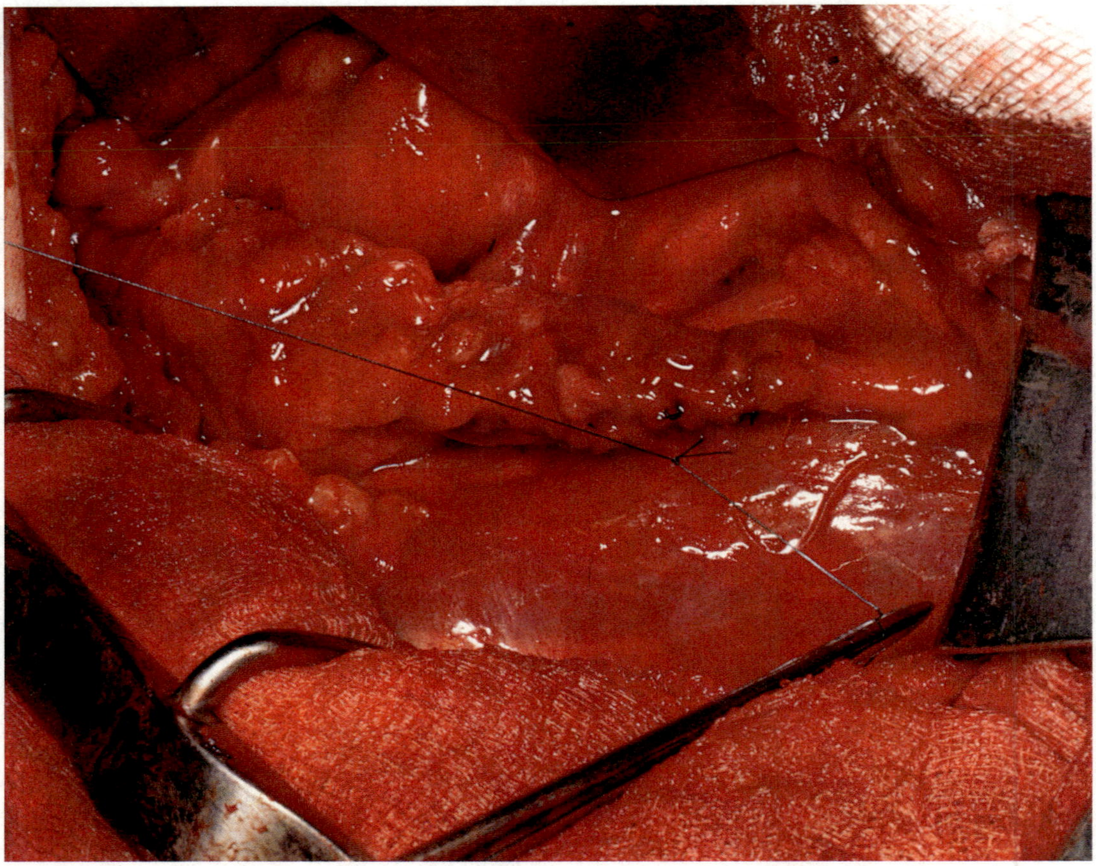

61 Completion of the suturing of the flap to the psoas muscle.

61

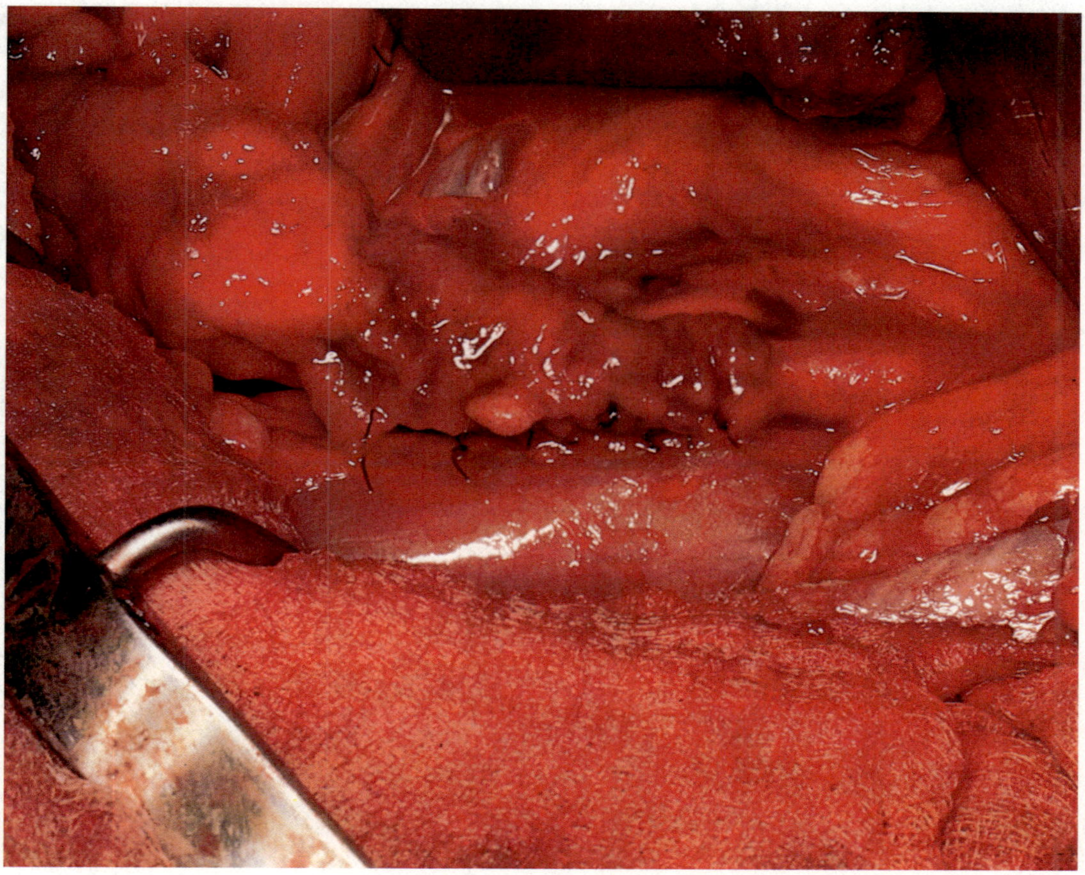

62 Finally, perivesical tissue is used to cover over the anastomosis, and also the incision of the flap down to the bladder.

62

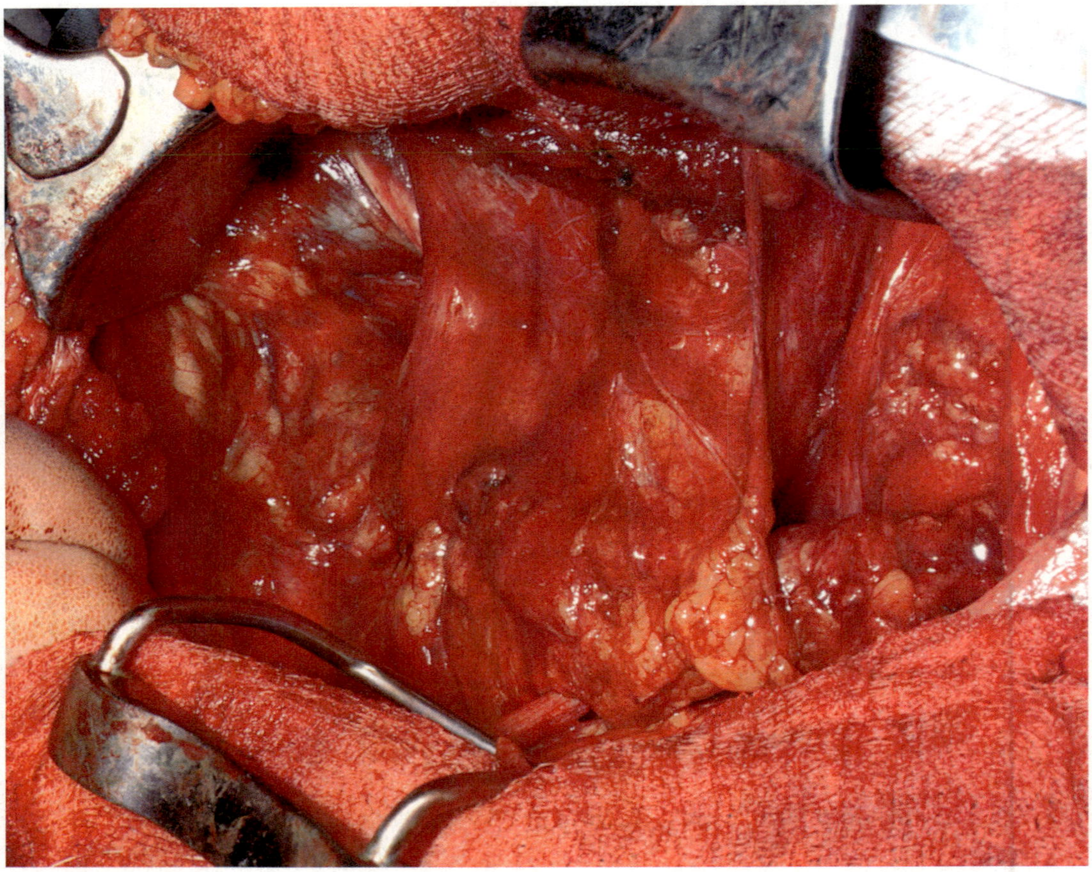

63

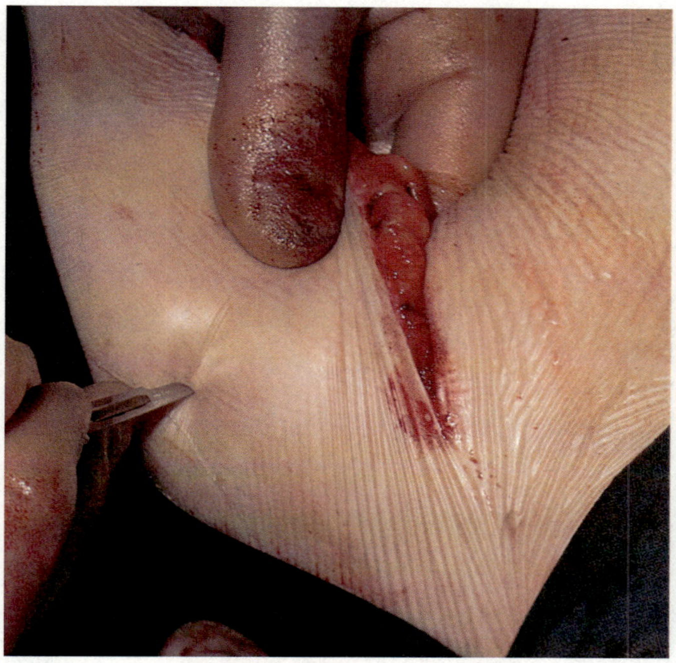

64

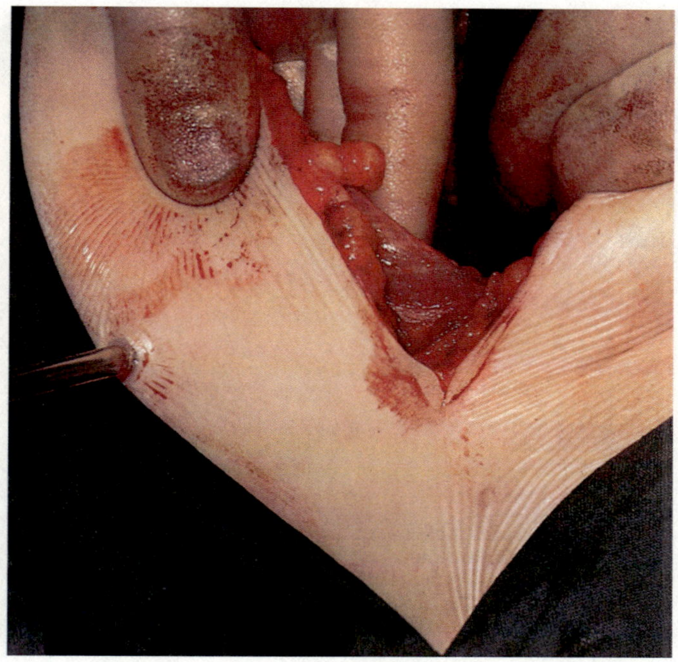

63 and 64 A drainage tube is inserted. The author prefers a simple low pressure suction drain.

65

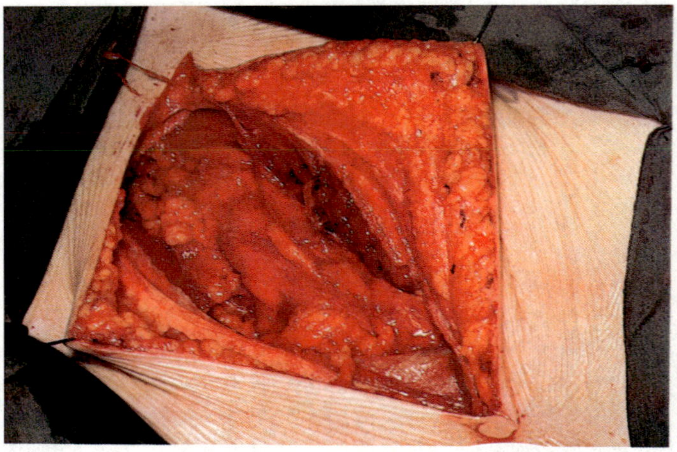

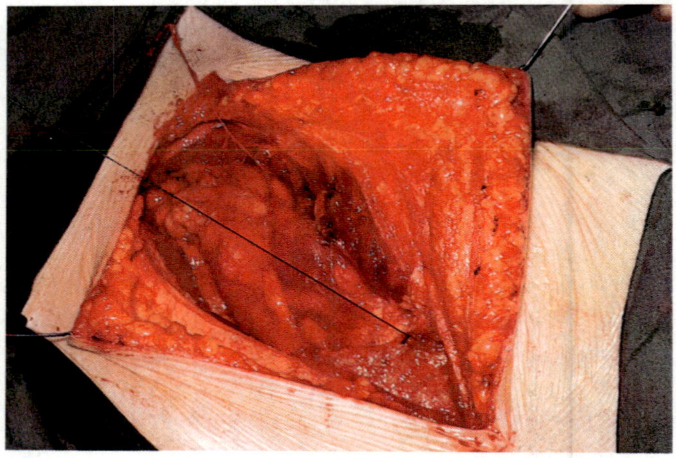

66

65 The wound is closed in layers using 0 Dexon continuous interlocking sutures, which is quite strong enough to close this incision. Interrupted sutures may be used, but muscle heals quickly, so the method of closure must remain the decision of the individual surgeon. Note again the use of skin hooks, and the excellent exposure.

66 Start of suturing transversalis and internal oblique.

67 Layer half closed.

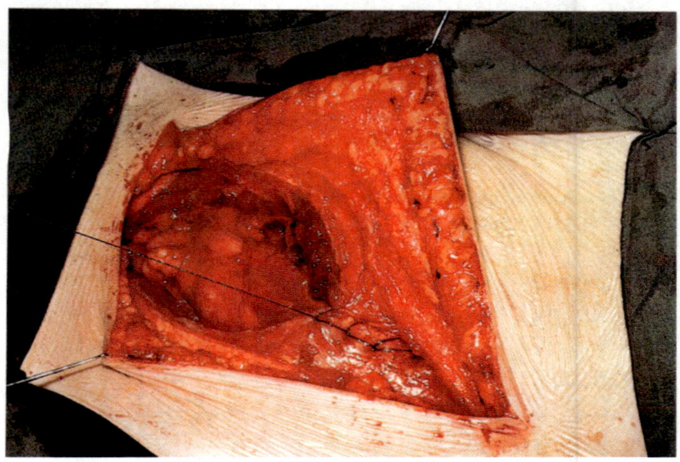

67

68

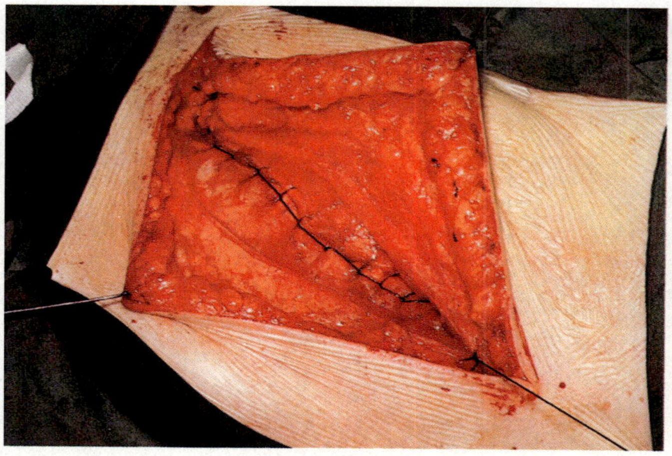

69

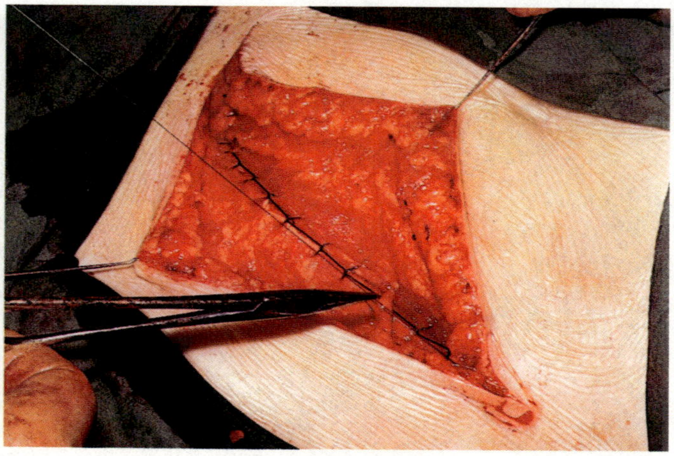

68 **Completion of the first layer of sutures.**

69 and 70 **Closure of the external oblique.**

70

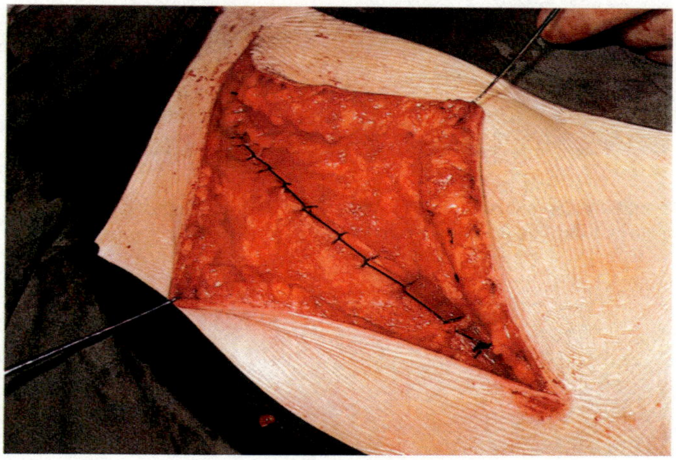

71

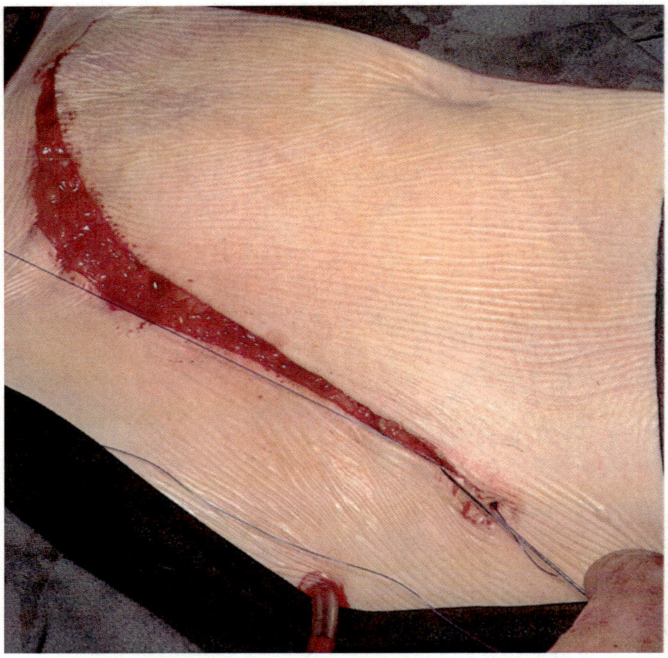

72

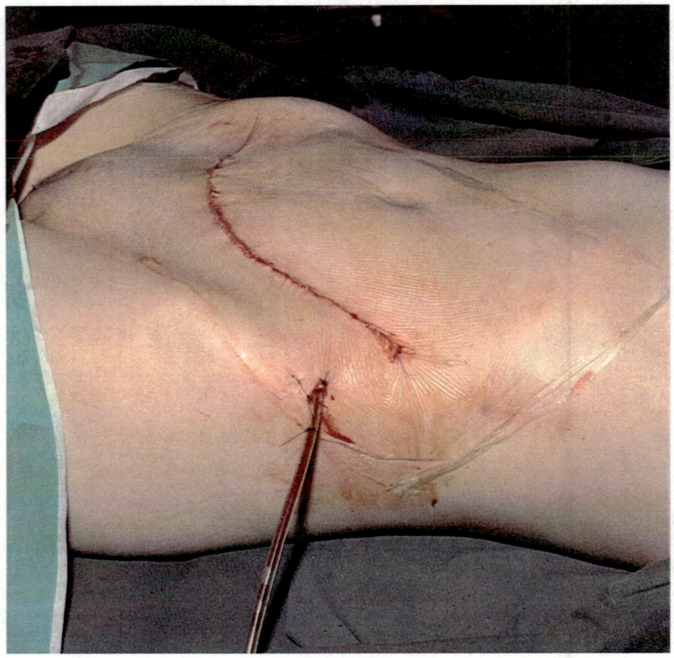

71 and 72 A subcuticular fat suture is also inserted, and the final closure of the skin is in a subcuticular 3.0 nylon.

73

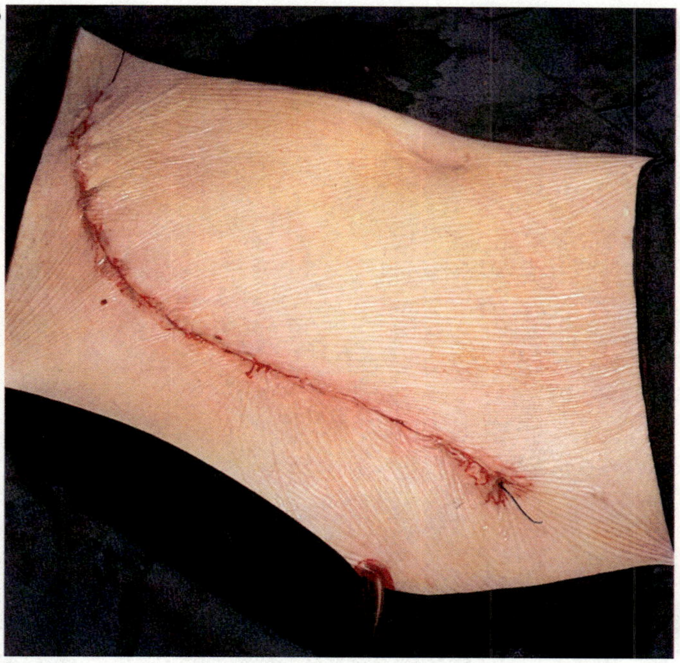

74

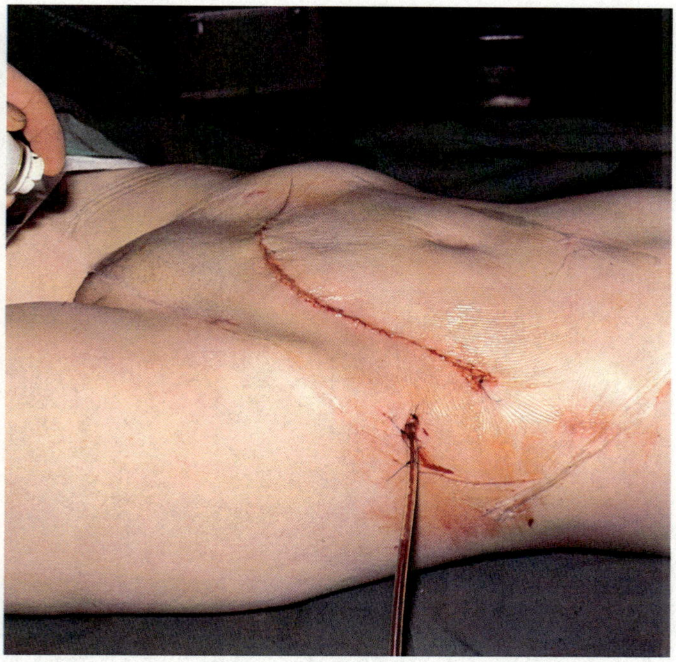

73 The Op-site is left on the skin for a period of four to five days.

74 The wound is sealed by spraying it with Op-site spray.

75

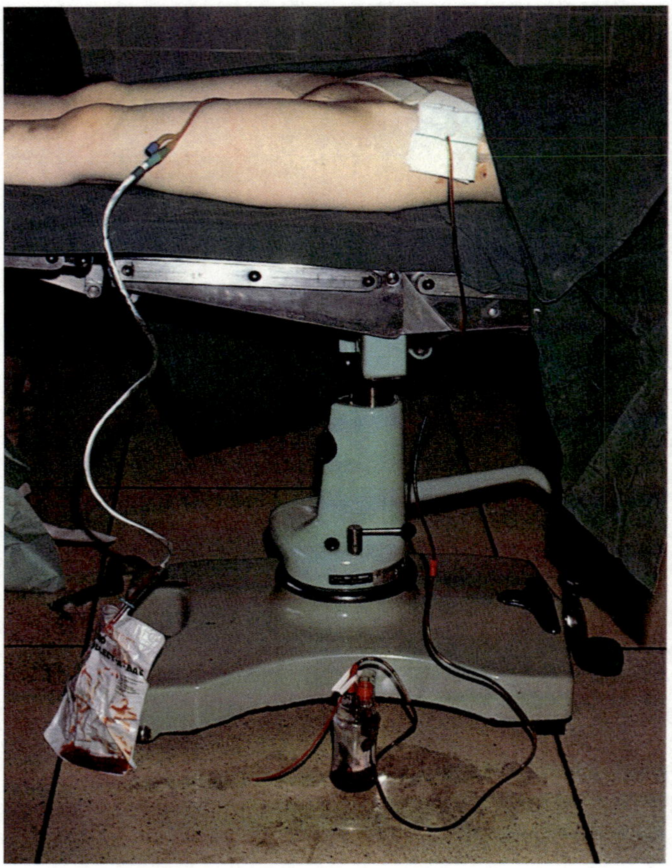

75 **The catheter is attached to a closed drainage system**, and suction is attached to the suction bottle.

76

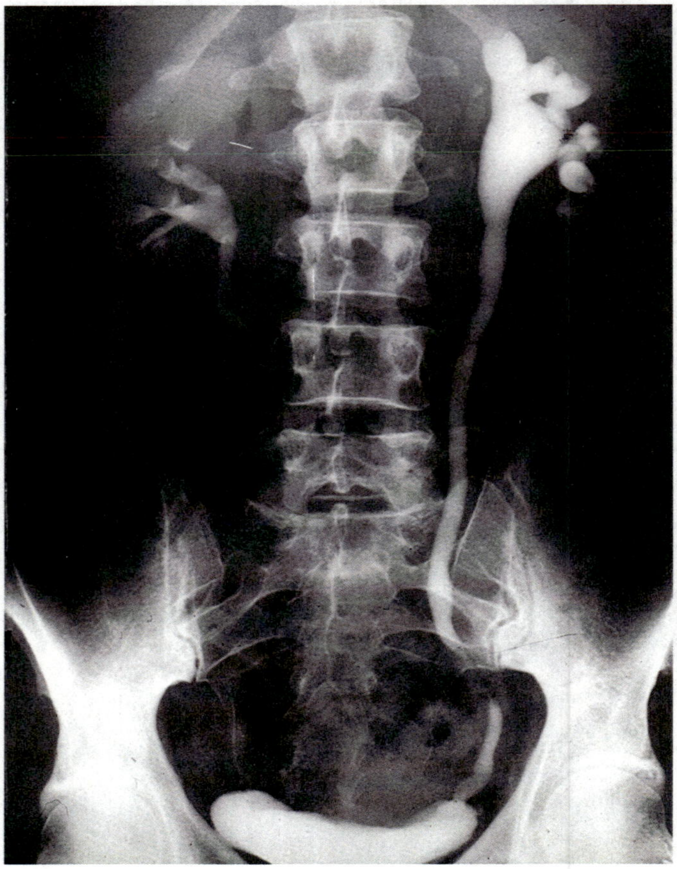

76 **Tuberculous hydronephrosis with early dilatation of the ureter.** A stricture about 5 cm in length is present at the lower end of the ureter.

77

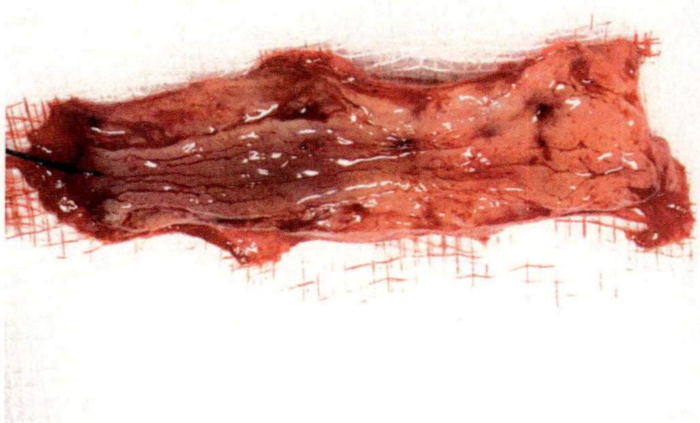

77 **Resected specimen showing the extent of the disease.**

78

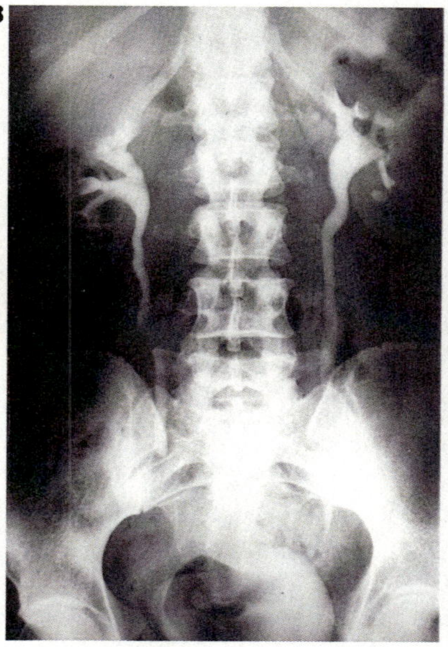

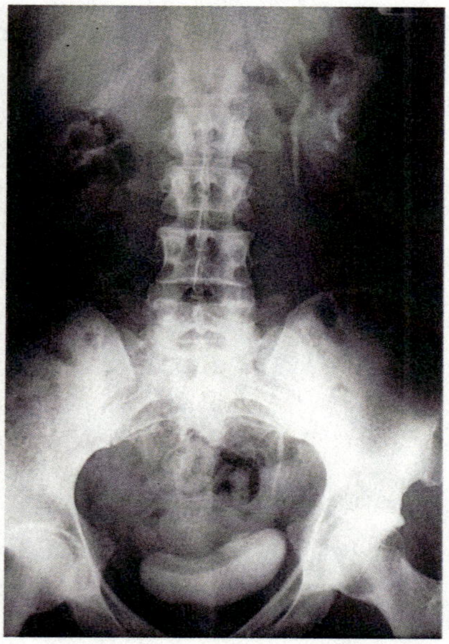

78 and 79 The result of Fig. 76 with a full and partially empty bladder. Note how the Boari flap conforms to the ureter and cannot be identified as part of the bladder.

References

Cukier, J., 1966, *Acta urol. Belg.* **34**, 15.

Gow, J.G., 1968. *Proc. R. Soc. Med.*, **61**, 128–130. The results of the reimplantation of the ureter by the Boari technique.

Konigsberg, H., Blunt, K.J. and Muecke, E.C., 1975. *Urology*, **V**, 6, 751–755. Use of Boari flap in lower ureteral injuries.

Thompson, I.M. and M.D., 1977. *Urological clinics of North America*. **4**, 1, 51–57.

Index

Numbers in medium type indicate page numbers; those in **bold** refer to figure and caption numbers.

FSC
www.fsc.org
MIX
Papier | Fördert
gute Waldnutzung
FSC® C083411

Kolibri 360 GmbH
Ferdinand-Jühlke-Straße 7
99095 Erfurt, Deutschland
produktsicherheit@kolibri360.de